Liver Failure

Guest Editors

DINESH YOGARATNAM, PharmD, BCPS
SARAH SAXER, PharmD
TENITA P. FOSTON, RN, MSN, FNP-C

CRITICAL CARE NURSING CLINICS OF NORTH AMERICA

www.ccnursing.theclinics.com

Consulting Editor
JANET FOSTER, PhD, RN, CNS

September 2010 • Volume 22 • Number 3

SAUNDERS an imprint of ELSEVIER, Inc.

W.B. SAUNDERS COMPANY
A Division of Elsevier Inc.

Elsevier Inc., 1600 John F. Kennedy Blvd., Suite 1800, Philadelphia, PA 19103-2899

http://www.theclinics.com

CRITICAL CARE NURSING CLINICS OF NORTH AMERICA Volume 22, Number 3
September 2010 ISSN 0899-5885, ISBN-13: 978-1-4377-1809-6

Editor: Katie Hartner

Critical Care Nursing Clinics of North America (ISSN 0899-5885) is published quarterly by Elsevier Inc., 360 Park Avenue South, New York, NY 10010-1710. Months of issue are March, June, September, and December. Business and Editorial Offices: 1600 John F. Kennedy Blvd., Suite 1800, Philadelphia, PA 19103-2899. Periodicals postage paid at New York, NY and additional mailing offices. Subscription prices are $130.00 per year for US individuals, $256.00 per year for US institutions, $68.00 per year for US students and residents, $167.00 per year for Canadian individuals, $321.00 per year for Canadian institutions, $191.00 per year for international individuals, $321.00 per year for international institutions and $99.00 per year for Canadian and foreign students/residents. To receive student/resident rate, orders must be accompanied by name of affiliated institution, data of term, and the *signature* of program/residency coordinator on institution letterhead. Orders will be billed at individual rate until proof of status is received. Foreign air speed delivery is included in all *Clinics* subscription prices. All prices are subject to change without notice. **POSTMASTER:** Send address changes to *Critical Care Nursing Clinics of North America*, Elsevier Health Sciences Division, Subscription Customer Service, 3251 Riverport Lane, Maryland Heights, MO 63043. **Customer Service: 1-800-654-2452 (US and Canada); 314-447-8871 (outside US and Canada). Fax: 314-447-8029. E-mail: JournalsCustomerService-usa@elsevier.com (for print support) and JournalsOnlineSupport-usa@elsevier.com (for online support).**

Reprints. For copies of 100 or more of articles in this publication, please contact the Commercial Reprints Department, Elsevier Inc., 360 Park Avenue South, New York, New York, 10010-1710; Tel.: (212) 633-3813, Fax: (212) 462-1935, and E-mail: reprints@elsevier.com.

Critical Care Nursing Clinics of North America is covered in *MEDLINE/PubMed (Index Medicus), International Nursing Index, Nursing Citation Index, Cumulative Index to Nursing and Allied Health Literature,* and *RNdex Top 100.*

Printed and bound in the United States of America
Transferred to Digital Print 2011

Contributors

CONSULTING EDITOR

JANET FOSTER, PhD, RN, CNS
Texas Woman's University, College of Nursing, Houston, Texas

GUEST EDITORS

DINESH YOGARATNAM, PharmD, BCPS
Clinical Pharmacy Specialist, UMass Memorial Medical Center, Worcester, Massachusetts

SARAH SAXER, PharmD
Clinical Pharmacy Specialist, Emory University Hospital, Atlanta, Georgia

TENITA P. FOSTON, RN, MSN, FNP-C
Family Nurse Practitioner, Emory University Hospital, Atlanta, Georgia

AUTHORS

AHMAD ABOU ABBASS, MD
Transplant Surgical Fellow, Division of Transplant, Henry Ford Hospital, Detroit, Michigan

WANDA ALLISON, RN, BSN, CCTC
Manager, Clinical Operations & Services, Emory Liver Transplant Program, Emory Healthcare, Atlanta, Georgia

DAVID CARPENTAR, MPAS, PA-C
Physician Assistant, Center for Critical Care, Emory Healthcare, Atlanta, Georgia

TRAM B. CAT, PharmD, BCPS
Clinical Pharmacy Specialist, Critical Care, Department of Pharmacy, Antelope Valley Hospital, Lancaster, California

JAMES N. FLEMING, PharmD, BCPS
Clinical Specialist, Solid Organ Transplant, Department of Pharmacy Services, Henry Ford Hospital, Detroit, Michigan

KEITH J. FOSTER, PharmD, BCPS
Clinical Pharmacist, Surgical Intensive Care Unit, Department of Pharmacy, UMass Memorial Medical Center, Worcester, Massachusetts

TENITA P. FOSTON, RN, MSN, FNP-C
Family Nurse Practitioner, Emory University Hospital, Atlanta, Georgia

AKIKO HATTORI, PharmD
Clinical Pharmacist, USC University Hospital, Los Angeles, California

JIWON W. KIM, PharmD, BCPS, FCSHP
Assistant Professor, Department of Clinical Pharmacy and Pharmaceutical Economics
and Policy, University of Southern California School of Pharmacy, USC University
Hospital, Los Angeles, California

ISHAQ LAT, PharmD
Clinical Coordinate - Clinical Pharmacist Specialist, Medical Intensive Care Unit,
Department of Pharmacy Services, University of Chicago Medical Center,
Chicago, Illinois

SONIA LIN, PharmD, BCPS
Clinical Associate Professor, Department of Pharmacy Practice, College of Pharmacy,
University of Rhode Island, Kingston, Rhode Island; Clinical Pharmacy Specialist (Solid
Organ Transplantation), Department of Pharmacy, UMass Memorial Medical Center,
Worcester, Massachusetts

XI LIU-DERYKE, PharmD
Trauma ICU Clinical Specialist, Department of Pharmacy, Orlando Regional Medical
Center, Orlando, Florida

G. MARSHALL LYON III, MD, MMSc
Assistant Professor of Medicine, Director of Transplant Infectious Diseases, Division
of Infectious Diseases, Emory University School of Medicine, Atlanta, Georgia

AMIT MAHAJAN, MD
Department of Medicine - Section of Pulmonary and Critical Care Medicine, University
of Chicago Medical Center, Chicago, Illinois

SHARON B. MATHEWS, MS, RN, CPTC
Clinical Manager, Transplant Services, UMass Memorial Medical Center, Worcester,
Massachusetts

ANEESH K. MEHTA, MD
Assistant Professor of Medicine, Assistant Director of Transplant Infectious Diseases,
Division of Infectious Diseases, Emory University School of Medicine, Atlanta, Georgia

PAULA V. PHONGSAMRAN, PharmD
Assistant Professor, Department of Clinical Pharmacy and Pharmaceutical Economics
and Policy, University of Southern California School of Pharmacy, USC University
Hospital, Los Angeles, California

PREETI A. RESHAMWALA, MD
Assistant Professor of Medicine, Digestive Diseases and Transplantation, Emory
University School of Medicine, Emory Healthcare, Atlanta, Georgia

BRIAN S. SMITH, PharmD, BCPS
Director, Education and Clinical Services, UMass Memorial Medical Center, Worcester,
Massachusetts

CHARLES J. TURCK, PharmD, BCPS
Clinical Pharmacy Specialist, Surgical Intensive Care Unit, Department of Pharmacy,
UMass Memorial Medical Center, Worcester, Massachusetts

VIVIAN M. ZHAO, PharmD, BCNSP
Clinical Pharmacist, Nutrition and Metabolic Support Service, Department
of Pharmaceutical Services, Emory University Hospital, Atlanta, Georgia

THOMAS R. ZIEGLER, MD
Attending Physician, Nutrition and Metabolic Support Service, Emory University Hospital;
Professor, Division of Endocrinology, Metabolism and Lipids, Department of Medicine,
Emory University School of Medicine; Atlanta Clinical & Translational Science Institute,
Emory University Hospital, Atlanta, Georgia

Contents

Patients with chronic liver diseases sustain impairment to immune systems, which worsens over time. These defects in their host defense lead
to risks of bacterial infections and increased morbidity. Providers should
have heightened surveillance for infectious diseases and suspect one
with any acute change in status. Patient history may reveal rare infections
and allow initiation of early appropriate therapy. There should be a low
threshold for obtaining diagnostic cultures and peritoneal fluid samples
and discussing possible causes with an infectious diseases consultant
or a microbiology laboratory. These maneuvers will maximize therapy in
patients at high risk for death due to infectious disease.

Ascites is the most common complication of cirrhosis, and it often leads to
hospitalization. Quality of life and mortality are negatively impacted by ascites. This article highlights the management of this potentially deadly
complication.

The depletion of vital coagulation factors and proteins in the setting of
acute liver failure (ALF) is common and multifactorial. The management
of critically ill patients with ALF is difficult and requires a multidisciplinary
approach to effective treatment. Critical care nurses are essential in identifying potential sources of bleeding, monitoring for transfusion reactions,
and staying vigilant for medication-related adverse reactions. Prevention
and treatment of bleeding disorders is a priority because ineffective therapy can lead to hazardous consequences. Correction of coagulopathy for
treatment of bleeding and reversal for invasive procedures should include
a multifactorial therapeutic plan emphasizing the correction of all coagulation factors. The limitations of current knowledge in effective correction
should serve as a stimulus for future research.

More than 1000 drugs have been associated with hepatic injury, which can
present in all forms of acute and chronic liver disease. The identification
and prevention of drug-induced liver disease remain challenging tasks

for health care professionals as reliable and practical assessment tools are not currently available to diagnose drug-induced liver disease. The management of drug-induced liver injury is generally supportive, and the recognition and avoidance of causative agents remain the most effective strategy for positive clinical outcomes.

Hepatic dysfunction in the critically ill patient presents a unique challenge to clinicians when designing pharmacotherapeutic treatment plans. Overall, the literature regarding drug dosing in critically ill patients with hepatic dysfunction is incomplete and current tools available to bedside clinicians have limitations. Despite these challenges, rational drug regimens can be implemented by critical care nurses who consider the potential impact of hepatic dysfunction on drug pharmacokinetics. This information can be applied clinically and careful monitoring plans can be implemented to assess a drug for efficacy and safety. This article reviews the pharmacokinetic changes that can occur in hepatic failure, identifies practical ways to quantify the severity of dysfunction, and discusses general drug dosing strategies in this patient population.

Hepatic encephalopathy (HE) is caused by liver impairment and has a multitude of symptoms in affected patients, including change in level of consciousness, intellectual function, and neuromuscular function. Pharmacologic therapy includes use of nonabsorbable disaccharides (lactulose and lactitol), and antibiotics such as neomycin, paromycin, metronidazole, and rifaximin. Probiotics, acarbose, and drugs such as L-carnitine and flumazenil, may also be helpful in treating HE.

Over the past 50 years, the pathophysiology and features of the hepatorenal syndrome have been illuminated. The syndrome can be divided into 2 distinct clinical patterns: a rapidly progressive renal failure with an extremely poor prognosis (type 1) and a slow progressive renal failure that correlates with the degree of cirrhosis (type 2). Although our understanding of hepatorenal syndrome continues to grow, our current methods of treating this condition remain limited in their effectiveness. The only definitive therapy is liver transplantation. This is a review of the definition, pathophysiology, and current recommendations for management of hepatorenal syndrome with the critical care nurse in mind.

Protein-calorie malnutrition is common in end-stage liver disease, irrespective of cause, and adversely affects clinical outcomes. Early diagnosis is important to allow appropriate intervention to prevent malnutrition-associated complications. Correction of nutrient deficiencies through oral supplementation, enteral tube feeding, or parenteral feeding can improve clinical outcomes in this patient population. This article addresses the causes of malnutrition, methods used to assess nutritional status, and treatment strategies in end-stage liver disease.

Tram B. Cat and Xi Liu-DeRyke

Gastroesophageal variceal hemorrhage is a major complication of portal hypertension in 50% to 60% of patients with liver cirrhosis and is a frequent cause of mortality in these patients. The prevalence of variceal hemorrhage is approximately 5% to 15% yearly, and early variceal rebleeding has a rate of occurrence of 30% to 40% within the first 6 weeks. More than 50% of patients who survive after the first bleeding episode will experience recurrent bleeding within 1 year. Management of gastroesophageal varices should include prevention of initial and recurrent bleeding episodes and control of active hemorrhage. Therapies used in the management of gastroesophageal variceal hemorrhage may include pharmacologic therapy (vasoactive agents, nonselective b-blockers, and antibiotic prophylaxis), endoscopic therapy, transjugular intrahepatic portosystemic shunt, and shunt surgery. This article focuses primarily on pharmacologic management of acute variceal hemorrhage.

Tenita P. Foston and David Carpentar

Acute liver failure (ALF) is an uncommon condition involving the rapid deterioration of liver functions and coagulation in previously well patients. The loss of liver function produces a cascade of systemic effects that rapidly overwhelm patients unless acted on. The key to managing patients with ALF revolves around having the resources and expertise to manage patients with rapidly evolving multiple system failure.

Sharon B. Mathews, Wanda Allison, and Sonia Lin

The detailed evaluation of a patient for liver transplant candidacy involves health care professionals from various disciplines to ensure that liver transplantation is optimal for patient morbidity and mortality from the medical and psychosocial perspective. The national liver allocation policy is complex and should be updated periodically based on continual assessment of outcomes that result from current policies. Streamlining of policies and procedures and implementing appropriate documentation across all transplant centers is required and regulated by National agencies such as OPTN/UNOS and CMS. This ensures safe and appropriate organ allocation and the delivery of high-quality transplant services.

THE CLINICS ARE NOW AVAILABLE ONLINE!
Access your subscription at:
www.theclinics.com

Preface

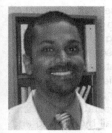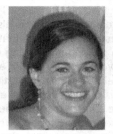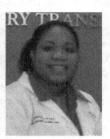

Dinesh Yogaratnam,   Sarah Saxer, PharmD   Tenita P. Foston,
    PharmD, BCPS   RN, MSN, FNP-C
                        Guest Editors

The liver is a complex organ responsible for myriad physiologic functions. Drug and toxin metabolism, protein synthesis, and glucose and nutrient regulation are just some of the crucial roles the liver plays in the human body. Not surprisingly, acute and chronic liver injury can lead to a plethora of both short-term and long-term adverse consequences. In this issue of *Critical Care Nursing Clinics of North America*, experts from a variety of disciplines discuss the challenges and controversies surrounding the care of the critically ill patient suffering from liver disease.

Acute liver disease portends a very poor prognosis. Foston provides an overview of this devastating disease state and touches on a variety of topics that are further elucidated in the other articles in this issue. Infectious complications as a result of chronic liver disease can result in significant morbidity. Mehta and Lyon describe the risk factors associated with infection and provide a detailed discussion on specific pathogens, sites of infection, and issues surrounding antibiotic selection. They also describe the role of vaccinations and the impact of infectious disease on transplant considerations.

Patients who are admitted to an intensive care unit will often require numerous medications during their acute illness. In the presence of liver disease, designing a pharmacotherapy regimen can become even more complicated. Lin and Smith discuss the consequences of altered liver function on the pharmacokinetics and pharmacodynamics of drugs. In addition, they provide general guidance on how to prospectively manage and evaluate drug therapy in the hepatically injured patient. Drug therapy can sometimes result in liver toxicity, which can occasionally be serious and fatal. Kim, Hattori, and Phongsamran discuss the epidemiology and risk factors associated with drug-induced liver disease. The pathophysiology associated with different toxic agents is discussed, and management and preventative strategies are put forth.

Nutritional support is a vitally important component in the management in liver disease. Inappropriate supplementation can increase the risk of complications, such as hepatic encephalopathy. Zhao and Ziegler provide an in-depth discussion on the many complex issues surrounding macro- and micronutrient support in liver disease.

Crit Care Nurs Clin N Am 22 (2010) xi–xii
doi:10.1016/j.ccell.2010.06.001   ccnursing.theclinics.com
0899-5885/10/$ – see front matter © 2010 Elsevier Inc. All rights reserved.

The liver is responsible for synthesizing coagulation factors. When damage to the liver occurs, coagulopathies may ensue. Mahajan and Lat describe the hemostatic complications associated with liver disease and provide a review of the many different therapies available to manage liver-related bleeding disorders. The acute reversal of coagulopathy, for the purposes of procedural interventions, is also discussed.

There are many unfortunate complications of liver disease that may require critical care services. Cat and Liu-DeRyke's article describes bleeding esophageal varices, a life-threatening complication of chronic liver disease. Treatment and preventative strategies for hepatic encephalopathy are elucidated in the article by Foster, Turk, and Lin. Reshamwala provides an overview of the strategies employed in treating abdominal ascites secondary to liver disease. One of the more devastating complications of liver disease, hepatorenal syndrome, is described in detail by Fleming and Abbass. Risk factors, epidemiology, and management strategies are described.

The definitive treatment for liver disease will sometimes be a liver transplant. The screening and approval process for liver transplantation has evolved significantly over the years. A thorough description of the contemporary transplant selection process is presented by Matthews, Allison, and Lin.

Dinesh Yogaratnam, PharmD, BCPS
UMass Memorial Medical Center
119 Belmont Street
Worcester, MA 01605, USA

Sarah Saxer, PharmD
Emory University Hospital
1364 Clifton Road, NE
Atlanta, GA 30322, USA

Tenita P. Foston, RN, MSN, FNP-C
Emory University Hospital
1364 Clifton Road NE
Atlanta, GA 30322, USA

E-mail addresses:
yogaratd@ummhc.org (D. Yogaratnam)
sarah.saxer@emoryhealthcare.org (S. Saxer)
Tenita.Foston@emoryhealthcare.org (T.P. Foston)

Infectious Diseases in End-Stage Liver Disease Patients

Aneesh K. Mehta, MD*, G. Marshall Lyon III, MD, MMSc

KEYWORDS

• Infection • Bacterial infections • Cirrhosis
• Sepsis • Spontaneous bacterial peritonitis

Patients with chronic liver dysfunction face a variety of immunologic impairments and microbiologic changes related to the underlying disease as well as the hepatic failure.[1] Infections in this group of patients may occur from these impairments or secondary to other complications of liver diseases and therapies. Bacterial infections are of particular concern in this patient population. Traditionally, patients with end-stage liver diseases (ESLDs) have high rates of spontaneous bacterial peritonitis (SBP), pneumonia, urinary tract infections, and sepsis, commonly due to community acquired gram-negative organisms.[2–4] Because the microbiology of communities and hospitals have changed, however, and the therapeutics and interventions have evolved, infections incurred by patients with hepatic dysfunction continue to challenge those who provide them care.

MECHANISMS OF INCREASED SUSCEPTIBILITY TO INFECTIOUS DISEASES
Altered Intestinal Permeability

Intact and functional mucosal immunity is vital to protecting humans against environmental and endogenous pathogens. Enteric flora are responsible for up to two-thirds of infections in ESLD.[4] Clinical and experimental data demonstrate that patients with cirrhosis develop diminished intestinal barriers, likely due to alterations in intracellular channels and cell integrity, leading to increased translocation of pathogens through the intestinal lining.[5,6] These translocated microorganisms enter the mesenteric and lymphatic circulatory systems and may disseminate from there. Furthermore, the bacterial endotoxins and antimicrobial responses lead to high levels of proinflammatory cytokines, regionally and systemically.[7] These processes may be amplified by concurrent alcohol use.[8] Prophylactic antibiotics, nonabsorbed and absorbed, may suppress intestinal bacterial, thereby decreasing the rate to translocation. Several

Division of Infectious Diseases, Emory University School of Medicine, Woodruff Memorial Research Building, Suite 2101, 101 Woodruff Circle, Atlanta, GA 30322, USA
* Corresponding author.
E-mail address: aneesh.mehta@emory.edu

Crit Care Nurs Clin N Am 22 (2010) 291–307
doi:10.1016/j.ccell.2010.04.002
0899-5885/10/$ – see front matter © 2010 Elsevier Inc. All rights reserved.

ccnursing.theclinics.com

therapeutic measures to decrease intestinal permeability to microbes in cirrhotic patients, including the use allopurinol, have not proved beneficial.[1]

Changes in Cytokine Profile

One of the most significant ramifications of bacterial translocation is the increased concentration of tumor necrosis factor α (TNF-α) and its inducible cytokines. TNF-α is vital component of hepatocyte injury response and usually promotes the proliferation of hepatocytes.[9] In the cirrhotic liver, however, the extent of hepatocyte injury leads to high levels of TNF-α, resulting in increased secretion of interleukin-1, interleukin-6, and interleukin-8 and activation of downstream kinases and proteases.[7] Thus, these adapted repair mechanisms are altered into a cycle that extends the hepatic damage, fibrosis, and cirrhois.[1]

Impaired Cellular Immunity

A large proportion of the immune dysfunction in cirrhotic patients occurs within the cellular immune system. Several groups have demonstrated that chronic hepatic dysfunction leads to neutrophil dysfunction, diminished activity of monocytes and macrophages, and reduced opsonification against pathogens.[10–14] All of these factors contribute to high rates of infections seen in this patient population; however, probably the most specific loss seen is within the reticuloendothelial system (RES). The RES is the primary defense system against pathogens in the blood and approximately 90% of these immune cells are located in the liver.[3] In cirrhosis, the RES activity is altered by two mechanisms: impairment of phagocytic activity of Kupffer cells (liver resident macrophages) and portosystemic shunting, leading to pathogens escaping exposure to the RES. This shunting and RES escape may also contribute to high levels of bacterial endotoxin and consequent changes in cytokine level (described previously).[15] Patients with a decreased RES activity are at higher risk of developing bacterial infections than patients with a normal RES.[16] As hepatic dysfunction worsens, the RES function continues to be lost and is largely responsible the higher rate of infections experienced in progressive cirrhosis.[4]

CLINICAL SYNDROMES AND ENTITIES

These immune system defects incurred with liver failure have a substantial clinical impact. Even in the era of broad-spectrum antibiotics, patients with cirrhosis have a high rate of bacterial infections, with a prevalence ranging from 32% to 44% in some studies.[2,4] The peritoneum, urinary tract, blood, and respiratory tract are the sites of the majority of these infections.[2,4] The majority of these infections develop in outpatients, but cirrhotic patients are also at increased risk for developing nosocomial infections given their frequent exposures and procedures.[2,17] Approximately two-thirds of community-derived infections are caused by enteric pathogens,[2,4] as expected with the underlying alterations in intestinal permeability. The severity and duration of cirrhosis seem to correlate to the risk of developing an infection.[4,17] Gastrointestinal hemorrhage has been established as significant risk factor for bacterial infections, but health care–related infections in particular are significantly higher in cirrhotic patients who present with bleeding.[4,17] Other parameters that confer increased risk of infection include low serum albumin, renal failure, serum bilirubin, and elevated white blood cell count at admission.[2,4,17] All but the last are likely a reflection of the severity of hepatic dysfunction. Although patients with cirrhosis are susceptible to all infections seen in the general population, certain infectious syndromes are more highly represented in this patient population than in others. These entities are discussed in this article.

Ascites and Spontaneous Bacterial Peritonitis

Approximately one-third of ESLD patients develop ascites, and 8% develop SBP. The clinical manifestations of SPB usually include fever, abdominal pain and tenderness, and altered mental status. These symptoms are neither specific nor sensitive for diagnosing SBP, however. A high index of suspicion is needed to appropriately diagnose SBP. Patients with cirrhosis often are hypothermic; therefore, anyone with a temperature above 37.8°C (100°F) should be evaluated for possible SBP. The diagnosis of SBP is based primarily on symptoms combined with analysis of the ascitic fluid. Paracentesis can be performed safely even in the setting of platelet dysfunction and elevated bleeding times often seen in ESLD. Ascitic fluid should be sent for cell count, culture, protein, lactate dehydrogenase (LDH), and glucose. A polymorphonuclear cell count of greater than 250 cells/mL supports the diagnosis of SBP. Elevated protein (>1 g/dL) or LDH combined with low glucose (<50 mg/dL) is concerning for bowel perforation; therefore, these patients should have imaging to assess for free, intraperitoneal air.

Bacterial translocation is the primary mechanism of SBP; therefore, most of the organisms causing disease are normal flora of the intestines, primarily *Escherichia coli* and *Klebsiella pneumoniae*. As such, antibiotic choices for treatment should adequately cover intestinal flora. Many antimicrobials have been evaluated. Oral fluoroquinolones (ciprofloxacin and levofloxacin) can be considered for patients who look relatively well. Intravenous therapy with cefotaxime was superior to ampicillin plus gentamicin. Therefore, cefotaxime or other similar third-generation cephalosporins are preferred for intravenous therapy. Penicillin plus β-lactamase inhibitor combinations as well as carbapenems have also been successfully used to treat SBP. Because many patients with ESLD often have renal impairment, antimicrobials should be appropriately adjusted for patients' renal function.

Because of the significant morbidity associated with SBP, many centers prefer to put ESLD patients with ascites on antimicrobial prophylaxis. A recent meta-analysis demonstrated that prophylaxis improved short-term survival and reduced the risk of infections, including SBP.[18] Therefore, antibiotic prophylaxis with a fluoroquinolones or trimethoprim-sulfamethosoxizole (TMP-SMX) should be considered for high-risk cirrhotic patients with ascites. Fluoroquinolones can be given weekly while patients are at risk, whereas TMP-SMX is often given as a single double-strength tablet once daily. Patients with moderate to severe renal impairment should have the dose of TMP-SMX reduced to a single-strength daily or a double-strength 3 times weekly.

Infections from Vibrio Species

Vibrio species are curved, gram-negative rods that are present in estuarine waters, where filter-feeding shellfish incorporate them into their normal microflora during the warmer months.[19] The best-known *Vibrio* species is *V cholerae*, which causes the feared epidemic diarrheal disease, cholera. The halophilic (salt-requiring) *Vibrio* species, however, *V parahaemolyticus* and *V vulnificus,* are of special interest for chronic liver disease patients. In the United States, *Vibrio*-related illnesses have seasonal peaks, with greater than 90% occurring between April and October.[19]

V parahaemolyticus was first identified in Japan, causing foodborne illnesses, and is now known to cause three clinical syndromes: gastroenteritis, wound infections, and septicemia.[20] Outbreaks in the United States generally are associated with consumption of raw or undercooked shellfish.[21] The vast majority of disease from this organism is a self-limited gastroenteritis, characterized by explosive watery diarrhea within 24 to 72 hours of ingestion and mild to moderately severe crampy abdominal pain.[19] Wound infections and bacteremia do occur, however.[19,20] In a Centers for Disease Control and Prevention (CDC) case series from the Gulf Coast Vibrio Surveillance system, 83% of sporadic *V parahaemolyticus* infections in those with liver disease developed septicemia, and overall mortality was 4%.[20]

The better-known halophilic *Vibrio* species, *V vulnificus*, is thought to have been first described by Hippocrates in the fifth century BC. This organism is found throughout the US Gulf Coast and parts of the Atlantic and Pacific coasts, residing in many shellfish species and some crabs during the warm summer months.[19,22] *V vulnificus* has evolved to have variety of virulence factors, including a capsular polysaccharide, acid neutralization, iron acquisition, and adhesion proteins, and is, therefore, more virulent than other noncholera *Vibrio* species.[19,23] These factors give *V vulnificus* a particular advantage in cirrhotic patients given the immune dysregulation (discussed previously), leading to an attributable risk of death of 38%.[22] Known risk factors for developing severe infections include cirrhosis, chronic hepatitis, alcohol abuse, diabetes, hemochromatosis, and chronic immunocompromised states as well as the consumption of raw or undercooked seafood.[22]

Infections from this organism are more often associated with a severe, distinctive soft tissue infection and septicemia, rather than a foodborne diarrheal disease.[19] In individuals with disturbed intestinal permeability, such as those with chronic liver disease, *V vulnificus* may invade into the bloodstream without causing gastrointestinal symptoms, inciting abrupt onset of fever and rigors. Symptoms progress often to development of metastatic cutaneous lesions and hypotension within 48 hours.[19] These cutaneous lesions may become bullous or necrotic and extend to develop myonecrosis as well. Liver disease patients who develop primary septicemia have a mortality rate ranging from 44% to 55%.[22–24]

In addition to septicemia, *V vulnificus* infections can result from direct inoculation leading to serious wound infections.[23] This situation usually occurs when a superficial wound becomes contaminated seawater containing *V vulnificus*. Direct tissue inoculation may occur also from fishing injuries, handling seafood, or trauma from contaminated materials.[22–24] Sinusitis, otitis, and ocular infection have also been reported.[19,22] A rapidly expanding cellulitis, necrotizing vasculitis, bullae formation, and ulcerative erosions may each or all develop from the site of inoculation.[19] Mortality from tissue-originated *V vulnificus* infections is approximately 25%.[23,24]

Diagnosis, treatment, and prevention of these *Vibrio* infections are similar. Practitioners caring for liver disease patients must have a heightened vigilance for these diseases. Stool cultures, wound cultures, or blood cultures should be collected in the appropriate settings. A microbiology laboratory needs to be informed of the potential diagnosis to actively search for and identify *Vibrio* spp. Limited gastroenteritis need not be treated in most patients; however, in cirrhotic, alcoholic, or immune-compromised patients with severe or progressive symptoms, antibiotics should be considered. Primary skin infections usually respond well to antibiotics if treated early.[19] Tissue disease from progressing wound infections or disseminated from septicemia often requires surgical débridement and amputation.[22,24] Bacteremic patients are often septic and in shock at presentation, and, therefore, require intravenous antibiotics plus early goal-directed resuscitation. Fluoroquinolones are the mainstay of antibiotic therapy; tetracycline class and third-generation cephalosporins may be used as well.[19] Good patient education and adherence can prevent many *Vibrio* infections. Patients with liver dysfunction should be advised, and periodically re-educated, not to eat raw or undercooked seafood. They should also be warned against swimming in brackish coast or estuarial waters or walking in coastal regions without appropriate protection. If they have open wounds or abrasions, they should avoid these activities altogether. Finally, patients should report any possible risk of exposure to a provider immediately, to ensure appropriate surveillance and early treatment if need.

Infections from Capnocytophaga Species

Capnocytophaga canimorsus (previous known as DF-2) is a thin gram-negative bacillus with tapered ends.[25] Infections from this organism are usually zoonotic, originating from the oral cavity dogs and cats in which *C canimorsus* is normal oral flora. Introduction of bacteria often occurs from penetrating traumas, such as a bite, or from inoculation through nonintact skin from saliva of the animal. Risk factors for invasive *C canimorsus* include asplenism and alcoholism.[26] Invasive disease resulting from such exposures is associated with high mortality rates and may manifest as sepsis, meningitis, endocarditis, or ocular infections.[27] The mortality rate for *C canimorsus* septicemia is approximately 25% to 33%, but mortality due to meningitis is much lower. *C canimorsus* sepsis manifestations are similar to other forms of gram-negative sepsis, although a prominent differential feature is the presence of a macular rash, found in 20% to 40% of cases.[25] This rash may progress to purpura fulminans, retiform purpura, or symmetric gangrene, which are often associated with disseminated intravascular coagulation and possibly Waterhouse-Friderichsen syndrome.[25,28,29]

Early diagnosis and therapy can positively influence outcomes. If the diagnosis is suspected, the practitioner should inform a microbiology laboratory of the concern. Blood and deep wound cultures should be obtained if possible. A presumptive diagnosis may be established if the characteristic slender, tapered, gram-negative rods are seen on a blood smear or blood culture smear. This organism is generally fastidious, however, and requires special techniques to be grown in culture.[25] Confirmatory testing usually requires a reference laboratory. Treatment starts with immediate débridement of the site to remove any foreign material, bacteria, and necrotic tissue. Once cultures and cleaning have started, it is often appropriate initiate empiric antibiotics; for most bites, amoxicillin-clavulanic acid is sufficient. Penicillin may be substituted once a diagnosis of *Capnocytophaga* is made; clindamycin and tetracycline class antibiotics are alternative for penicillin-allergic patients.[29] If a patient is presenting with sepsis, however, intravenous antibiotics with a β-lactam/β-lactase inhibitor or a carbapenem should be initiated. Patients with chronic liver disease should be advised not to allow pets to bite them, even in play, or lick opened skin areas, to prevent these types of infections.

Infections from Yersinia Enterocolitica

Yersinia enterocolitica is a facultatively anaerobic, oxidase-negative, gram-negative rod that can often appear pleomorphic in culture. Although most frequently encountered as a cause of bacterial enterocolitis in healthy people, this organism has a propensity to spread beyond the gastrointestinal tract in patients who are immunosuppressed, with chronic iron overload, or who are receiving deferoxamine and in those with chronic liver disease.[30,31] Bacteremia and sepsis are the most common complications of *Y enterocolitica* in this patient population, but metastatic diseases, such as liver abscesses, splenic abscesses, endocarditis, and osteomyelitis, may occur as well.[30] *Y enterocolitica* is a rare, but significant cause of SBP also. This entity has been exclusively reported in adults with ascites secondary to cirrhosis or hemochromatosis and has a 50% mortality rate.[32] Infections from *Y enterocolitica* often lead to postinfectious autoimmune processes, such as reactive arthritis, Reiter syndrome, erythema nodosum, and glomerulonephritis. Patients who are HLA-B27 positive are thought at greatest risk for developing these sequelae.[30] Treatment is not recommended for immunocompetent patients, but for those with immunocompromised states, such as cirrhosis, dual-agent therapy with doxycycline, TMP-SMZ, fluoroquinolone, or an aminoglycoside is recommended.[33]

Infections from Aeromonas Species

Aeromonads are heterotrophic, facultative anaerobic, gram-negative bacilli that are ubiquitous in fresh, estuarine, and brackish water bodies and occasionally contaminate potable water supplies.[34] Three species are known to cause disease in humans: A hydrophila, A caviae, and A veronii biovar sobria. Although Aeromonas bacteremias and sepsis are uncommon, the larger series reported in the literature have pointed to chronic liver diseases as the predominate predisposing diseases leading to this infection.[34–36] Almost half of these patients have a concomitant focus of infection, such as peritonitis, cellulitis, necrotizing fasciitis, cholangitis, or burns.[35] These invasive Aeromonas infection result in a 39% mortality rate.[35] More recently, Aeromonas has been found a highly prevalent cause of SBP in chronic liver disease patients, especially in Eastern Asia.[37,38] The incidence of Aeromonas SBP was found higher in warm months and when the presentation of SBP included diarrhea.[37] Despite early adequate antibiotics, Aeromonas SBP is associated with mortality rates between 23% and 56%.[37,38] Therefore, invasive Aeromonas infections are often fatal and must be considered in the differential diagnosis of patients with advanced liver cirrhosis in endemic areas and high-risk exposure.

The relevant Aeromonas species are resistant to penicillin and ampicillin and are often resistant to first- and second-generation cephalosporins, including cefotaxime. Obtaining antibiotic sensitivities from a microbiology laboratory is important to achieving the best therapy; however, most isoloates are susceptible to third-generation cephalosporins, aztreonam, and carbapenems.[34] Aeromonas spp have recently demonstrated the ability to produce a variety of resistant factors, including carbapenemases, and may develop resistance on therapy. Therefore, it is advisable to obtain an infectious disease consultation to determine optimal therapy in high-risk patients.

Infections from Listeria Monocytogenes

Listeria monocytogenes is motile, gram-positive, facultative, anaerobic bacillus that is found in contaminated water sources and animal products. This pathogen is well known to cause severe infections in patients with impaired cell-mediated immunity, including neonates, pregnant women, patients with AIDS, elderly persons, chemotherapy recipients, and transplant recipients. L monocytogenes has also become recognized as an important cause of SBP in advanced cirrhosis, with almost 40 cases in the literature.[39,40] Listeria SBP is especially prevalent in those with comorbidities, such as diabetes mellitus, cancer, and HIV.[40] Concomitant bacteremia is frequently present, and development of meningitis is possible.[40] Overall mortality rate is approximately 30% from Listeria SBP.[40]

Ampicillin is generally the preferred agent for all forms of listeriosis. TMP-SMX is thought the best alternative for those with a penicillin allergy. Carbapenems, fluoroquinolones, and vancomycin are possible alternatives, but there are limited human data for these agents.[41] Combination therapy with ampicillin plus TMP-SMX may have better outcomes than monotherapy.[42] Meningitis dosing should be used for all patients, even in the absence of neurologic abnormalities, because of L monocytogenes' predilection for the central nervous system.

Bacteremia and Sepsis

Patients with hepatic dysfunction have an increased risk for bacteremia and sepsis.[15] As discussed previously, bacteria may enter the bloodstream by multiple mechanisms and may quickly progress to sepsis and multiorgan failure due to the immune dysfunctions occurring in cirrhotic patients. Although bacteremia may occur secondary to a pre-existing infection or recent instrumentation, this group of patients often develops spontaneous bacteremia. Many of these cases may be incited by occult or overt gastrointestinal bleeding, which is known to greatly increase the risk of bacterial infections.[17] A recent Cochrane Database review found that the accumulated data in eight trials demonstrated that antibiotic prophylaxis at time of gastrointestinal hemorrhage had a significant benefit by decreasing mortality and the incidence of bacterial infections.[43] Despite general adoption of bacterial prophylaxis, cirrhotic patients still have a high rate of bacterial diseases, which often progress to sepsis and severe sepsis. The mechanisms for this progression, and the organ damage that results, has been nicely reviewed recently.[44]

Foreman and colleagues[45] evaluated the National Hospital Discharge Survey to determine the impact of concurrent hepatic failure and sepsis. Cirrhotic patients were more likely to develop sepsis during admission than those without cirrhosis, 4.6% versus 1.9%, respectively.[45] In particular, these investigators found that patients with cirrhosis were 3.5 times more likely than noncirrhotic patients to have gram-positive infections and 2.8 times more likely to have gram-negative infections during a hospital admission.[45] The adjusted relative risk for death due sepsis for patients with hepatic failure was 2.0.[45]

Given the degree of immune dysfunction and the morbidity of infections, patients with significant cirrhosis who present with, or with probable, bacteremia or sepsis should undergo rapid diagnostic testing and should receive intravenous antibiotics that treat the likely organisms as soon as possible. In septic patients, early antibiotic initiation with the appropriate agents significantly improves outcomes,[46,47] and this effect is especially important in immunocompromised patients. If patients have been recently treated with or are on prophylaxis with a fluoroquinolone, it is prudent to not depend on this class. Given the high prevalence of gram-negative bacterial etiology, however, broad coverage of these organisms is needed. Therefore, piperacillin/tazobactam and ceftazidime are appropriate empiric agents covering most enteric organisms as well as *Pseudomonas* spp, *Vibrio* spp, and *Capnocytophaga* spp. If patients are presenting with a community-acquired pneumonia and do not meet criteria for a health care–associated pneumonia, then it is reasonable to initiate an β-lactam (ceftriaxone, cefotaxime, or ampicillin-sulbactam) plus a macrolide. If patients have an indwelling catheter, port, or drain, and there is a significant prevalence of methicillin-resistant *Staphylococcus aureus* (MRSA) in the community, vancomycin may be added. Cirrhotic patients with previous significant antibiotic exposure or fluoroquinolone prophylaxis increase the rates of carriage of resistant gram-negatives and MRSA and may be associated with increased infections with MRSA.[48] Rapid initiation of diagnostic tests is paramount to achieving a definitive diagnosis. Complete blood count, renal function test, liver function tests, and blood cultures are generally necessary for all cirrhotic patients presenting with possible sepsis. Symptom-directed radiographs, diagnostic paracentesis (if ascites present), urine analysis with microscopy (if urinary tract symptoms present), and sputum cultures (if respiratory symptoms present) are often needed. If certain risk factors, such as raw seafood exposure or animal bites, are perceived, additional special cultures or tests may be needed. As with any severely ill patient, the results of these tests need to be carefully interpreted in context with patients' progress.

INFECTIOUS DISEASES MANAGEMENT ISSUES
Antimicrobial Agents

Because the liver plays a central role in the metabolism and clearance of several anti-infective agents, hepatic dysfunction and subsequent changes in hepatic enzymes, biliary excretion, protein binding, and portal-systemic shunting may lead to modified pharmacokinetics and pharmacodynamics of these drugs. Although many of these alterations may not be clinically significant, those drugs that need dosage adjustment for hepatic dysfunction are summarized in **Table 1.** Liver diseases are common in patients infected with HIV, and these patients required special attention. Cirrhosis and hepatic failure, however, are not contraindications to highly active antiretroviral therapy, which substantially reduces the risk of liver-related mortality in these patients.[49] The recommendations for antiretrovirals (listed in **Table 1**) should be made in consultation with an expert HIV provider.

Probiotics

Recent research in the use of certain probiotic agents has shown promise in decreasing cytokine release and improving neutrophil function in cirrhotic patients.[50,51] There are no data to support decreasing infection rates or improved outcomes with probiotics in this population, however. Furthermore, a recent randomized clinical trial of probiotics in patients with severe acute pancreatitis resulted in an increased 90-day mortality; therefore, probiotics should not be used outside the research setting at this juncture.[52,53]

Vaccinations

Much of the care of patients with cirrhosis is focused on the diminishing further insult to the liver. Appropriate vaccination is an important component of this aspect of care. Vaccination against hepatitis A and B can help prevent a superimposed injury or fulminant hepatic failure to a liver that has little reserve. Both these vaccination series are recommended for all chronic liver diseases patients by the Advisory Committee on Immunization Practices and the CDC.[54] Given high rates of bacterial pneumonia and poor outcomes with pneumococcal sepsis in cirrhotic patients, pneumococcal polysaccharide vaccination is also recommended for this group.[54]

No commonly used vaccines are contraindicated by hepatic failure alone. Therefore, pneumococcal vaccine and yearly influenza vaccination should also be considered.

Screening End-Stage Liver Disease Patients for Transplantation

Organ transplantation has become the preferred, definitive treatment of ESLD. As a result of increasingly intense immunosuppressive regimens to reduce organ rejection, infections are becoming increasingly problematic in transplant recipients. With careful pretransplant screening, however, many infectious complications can be mitigated or eliminated altogether. There have been many pathogens that have been transmitted from organ donor to recipient or have reactivated in a recipient after transplantation due to immunosuppression—these are listed in **Box 1**. Currently, the United Network for Organ Sharing requests, but does not require, the following recipient serologies: HIV, cytomegalovirus (CMV), Epstein-Barr virus, hepatitis B virus, and hepatitis C virus. Many transplant centers also test for many infections, however, which may be latent and become manifest after initiation of immunosuppression. Tests that are commonly used for pretransplantation screening are listed in **Box 2**.

Table 1
Summary of antimicrobial agents for which dosage adjustment may be considered for hepatic dysfunction

Drug	Dosing Adjustment
Antibacterials	
Ceftriaxone	Not to exceed 2 g daily, if hepatic AND renal dysfunction coexist
Clindamycin	Should not given more frequently than every 8 hours
Isoniazid	Contraindicated in acute hepatic injury or history of previous isoniazid-related hepatic dysfunction
Metronidazole	May need decreased dosage with long-term use in patients with severe hepatic impairment
Nafcillin	Serum nafcillin levels monitoring for patients with hepatic insufficiency and renal failure
Quinupristin/ dalfopristine	May need decreased dosage with long-term use in patients with Child-Pugh score >9
Tigecycline	In patients with Child-Pugh score >9, the maintenance dose should be reduced to 25 mg every 12 hours
Antifungals	
Caspofungin	In patients with Child-Pugh score 7–9, reduced maintenance dose to 35 mg daily; there are no data in patients with Child-Pugh score >9
Itraconazole	Relative contraindication in moderate to severe hepatic impairment
Voriconazole	In patients with Child-Pugh score 5–9, reduced maintenance dose by 50%; there are no data in patients with Child-Pugh score >9
Antivirals	
Abacavir	Child-Pugh score 5–6, 200 mg BID; >6, contraindicated
Nevirapine	Child-Pugh class >6, contraindicated
Atazanavir	Child-Pugh score 7–9, 300 mg once daily; >9 not recommended; boosting is not recommended in patients with Child-Pugh score >7
Darunavir	Not recommended in severe hepatic impairment
Fosamprenavir	Dose adjustments required if Child-Pugh >4, dose dependent on situation; please see reference
Indinavir	600 mg q8h for mild to moderate hepatic insufficiency; 200 mg BID if boosted
Nelfinavir	Not recommended in moderate to severe hepatic impairment
Saquinavir	Use with caution in mild to moderate hepatic impairment; contraindicated in severe hepatic impairment:
Tipranavir	Contraindicated in Child-Pugh score >6

Data from Refs.[71–73]

Obtaining a positive result on any of these serologic tests does not necessarily exclude a patient from receiving an organ. It does allow, however, for expectant management or prevention of infection or acute disease. For instance, knowing that a patient is serologically negative for CMV but will be receiving an organ from a serologically positive donor allows for the administration of prophylactic ganciclovir. Oral ganciclovir has been shown to effectively reduce CMV infection after solid organ transplant.[55–57] Similarly, recently published guidelines on TB in transplantation recommend, if feasible, to treat PPD-positive patients with isoniazid prior to transplantation.[58] In this way, significant morbidity and mortality can be avoided in a transplant

---

Box 1
Pathogens with transmission through solid-organ donation

Bacteria

Bacteremias

Bacterial meningitis (*Neisseria meningitidis*)

Staphylococcus aureus

Klebsiella species

Bacteroides species

Pseudomonas species

Listeria monocytogenes

Rickettsia rickettsii

Treponema pallidum

Legionella species

Brucella species

Bartonella species

Enterobacter species

Acinetobacter species

Viruses

CMV

Varicella zoster virus

HSV 1 and herpes simplex virus 2

EBV

Human herpesvirus 6

Human herpesvirus 7

Human herpesvirus 8 (Kaposi sarcoma–associated herpesvirus)

Hepatitis B

Hepatitis C

HIV

TLV

Rabies

Parvovirus B19

West Nile virus

BK virus

Lymphocytic choriomeningitis virus

Influenza A

Fungi

Aspergillus species

Candida species (candidemia)

Coccidioides immitis/podasii

Cryptococcus neoformans

Histoplasma capsulatum

Scedosporium apiospermum

Agents of mucormycosis (zygomycosis)

Prototheca species

Mycobacteria

Mycobacterium tuberculosis

Nontuberculous mycobacteria

Parasites

Toxoplasma gondii

Trypanosoma cruzi

Schistosomiasis

Strongyloides stercoralis

Plasmodium species (malaria)

Abbreviations: CMV, cytomegalovirus; EBV, epstein-Barr virus; HSV, herpes simplex virus; TLV, T-cell lymphotrophic virus.
Data from Rimola A, Soto R, Bory F et al. Reticuloendothelial system phagocytic activity in cirrhosis and its relation to bacterial infections and prognosis. Hepatology 1984;4(1):53–8; Deschenes M, Villeneuve J-P. Risk factors for the development of bacterial infections in hospitalized patients with cirrhosis. Am J Gastroenterol 1999;94(8):2193–7.

Box 2
Serologic tests used to evaluate solid-organ transplant candidates

UNOS requested

    HIV antibody

    CMV antibodies

    Epstein-Barr virus antibodies

    Hepatitis B surface antigen, surface antibody, core antibody

    Hepatitis C antibody

Commonly obtained additional serologic or screening tests

    Herpes simplex virus antibodies

    Varicella zoster virus antibodies

    Toxoplasma antibody

    Rapid plasma reagin (syphilis)

    Purified protein derivative (PPD) of tuberculosis (TB) or IGRA for TB

    Human T-cell lymphotrophic virus (HTLV-1 or HTLV-2) antibody

    Strongyloides

    Trypanososoma cruzi antibodies (for patients from endemic areas)

    Coccidioides antibodies (for patients from endemic areas)

Data from Fischer SA, Avery RK. Screening of donor and recipient prior to solid organ transplantation. Am J Transplant 2009;9(Suppl 4):S7–18.

recipient. Unfortunately, because TB treatments are sometimes hepatotoxic, it may not be feasible to treat ESLD patients prior to transplant.

For TB screening, the PPD has been traditionally used to screen for TB. Although effective, it is sometimes inconvenient for evaluating patients who live far from a medical center. After the PPD is placed, the patient must return in 48 to 72 hours to have the PPD interpreted. Thus, the patient makes a long-distance trip twice in quick succession, something that many ESLD patients may not tolerate well. Additionally, interpreting the PPD can be problematic because untrained health care workers often measure erythema rather than induration. Also, there are different cutoff points for different populations—15 mm for the general population, 10 mm for at-risk persons (health care workers and immigrants from endemic areas), and 5 mm for high-risk persons (those with recent exposure or who are immunocompromised). National guidelines recommend using 5 mm of induration for patients being considered for transplantation.[58] In the past few years, an alternative to PPD testing has emerged. These are interferon-gamma release assays (IGRAs). These tests simplify TB testing because they are blood tests and require only a single contact with a patient. In addition, unlike the PPD, which is subject to interpretation bias, IGRAs are machine read and have single cutoffs. Thus, there is little subjectivity to the reading of results. IGRAs have been tested and found to perform reasonably well in healthy populations[59,60] and in end-stage renal disease,[61,62] ESLD,[63] and other immunocompromised patients.[64–66]

In the past, HIV infection has been considered a contraindication to liver transplantation. Preliminary data from an ongoing multicentered study of the feasibility of liver transplantation in HIV-infected persons have shown, however, that outcomes are reasonable.[67] Of the first 11 patients enrolled, the 1-year survival in liver transplants was 91%.[67] This compares with 88.6% 1-year survival nationally in all liver transplant recipients.[68] HIV patients included in the study were highly selected, with well-controlled HIV.[67] Of the serologies listed in **Box 2**, many can be treated prior to transplantation, thus eliminating or greatly reducing the chance of active disease post transplant.

A reactive rapid plasma reagin should be treated with penicillin if not treated previously. Similarly, patients with evidence of Strongyloides or Trypanosoma infection should be treated prior to transplant. Strongyloides can be treated with a single dose of ivermectin. Ideally, patients should be managed with the assistance of an infectious diseases specialist. Treatment failures do occur with ivermectin so serology and blood counts need to be followed for resolution before transplant. Patients who test positive for hepatitis B or C, if not already done, should have additional testing performed to see if they have a chronic infection with either virus. If chronic infection is found, then consideration should be given to treating the chronic HBV or HCV infection, if not already attempted. If serology for herpes simplex viruses or varicella zoster virus is positive, these can be prevented by administration of acyclovir or valacyclovir after transplant. Similar to HIV, HTLV is not an absolute contraindication to receiving an organ transplant. In a kidney transplant series from Japan, there were no reactivations among 10 patients. Therefore, HTLV does not exclude someone from liver transplant.[69] A positive serology for an endemic fungus, especially Coccidioides, may require lifelong antifungal prophylaxis.[70]

SUMMARY

Patients with chronic liver diseases sustain impairment to their immune systems, which worsens over time and with disease progression. These defects in their host defense lead to augmented risks of bacterial infections and increased morbidity when they are incurred. Providers caring for patients with hepatic dysfunction should have a heighten surveillance for infectious diseases and suspect that one is present with any acute change in a patient's status. Careful elicitation of patient history and exposures may reveal rare but important infections and allow initiation of early appropriate therapy. In this patient population, there should be a low threshold for obtaining diagnostic cultures and peritoneal fluid samples as well as discussing possible causes with an infectious diseases consultant or a microbiology laboratory. These maneuvers maximize therapy in these patients at high risk for death due to infectious disease.

REFERENCES

1. Chavez-Tapia NC, Torre-Delgadillo A, Tellez-Avila FI, et al. The molecular basis of susceptibility to infection in liver cirrhosis. Curr Med Chem 2007;14(28): 2954–8.
2. Caly WR, Strauss E. A prospective study of bacterial infections in patients with cirrhosis. J Hepatol 1993;18(3):353–8.
3. Navasa M. Bacterial infections in patients with cirrhosis: reasons, comments and suggestions. Dig Liver Dis 2001;33(1):9–12.
4. Borzio M, Salerno F, Piantoni L, et al. Bacterial infection in patients with advanced cirrhosis: a multicentre prospective study. Dig Liver Dis 2001;33(1):41–8.
5. Campillo B, Pernet P, Bories PN, et al. Intestinal permeability in liver cirrhosis: relationship with severe septic complications. Eur J Gastroenterol Hepatol 1999;11(7):755–9.
6. Liu H, Zhang S, Yu A, et al. Studies on intestinal permeability of cirrhotic patients by analysis lactulose and mannitol in urine with HPLC/RID/MS. Bioorg Med Chem Lett 2004;14(9):2339–44.
7. Tilg H, Diehl AM. Cytokines in alcoholic and nonalcoholic steatohepatitis. N Engl J Med 2000;343(20):1467–76.
8. Fukui H, Brauner B, Bode JC, et al. Plasma endotoxin concentrations in patients with alcoholic and non-alcoholic liver disease: reevaluation with an improved chromogenic assay. J Hepatol 1991;12(2):162–9.
9. Diehl AM, Yin M, Fleckenstein J, et al. Tumor necrosis factor-alpha induces c-jun during the regenerative response to liver injury. Am J Physiol Gastrointest Liver Physiol 1994;267(4):G552–61.
10. Rajkovic IA, Williams R. Abnormalities of neutrophil phagocytosis, intracellular killing and metabolic activity in alcoholic cirrhosis and hepatitis. Hepatology 1986;6(2):252–62.
11. Clapperton M, Rolando N, Sandoval L, et al. Neutrophil superoxide and hydrogen peroxide production in patients with acute liver failure. Eur J Clin Invest 1997; 27(2):164–8.
12. Gomez F, Ruiz P, Schreiber AD. Impaired function of macrophage Fc gamma receptors and bacterial infection in alcoholic cirrhosis. N Engl J Med 1994; 331(17):1122–8.
13. Guarner C, Runyon BA. Macrophage function in cirrhosis and the risk of bacterial infection. Hepatology 1995;22(1):367–9.
14. Runyon BA. Patients with deficient ascitic fluid opsonic activity are predisposed to spontaneous bacterial peritonitis. Hepatology 1988;8(3):632–5 [Erratum appears in Hepatology 1988 Sep-Oct;8(5):1184].

15. Tandon P, Garcia-Tsao G. Bacterial infections, sepsis, and multiorgan failure in cirrhosis. Semin Liver Dis 2008;28(1):26–42.
16. Rimola A, Soto R, Bory F, et al. Reticuloendothelial system phagocytic activity in cirrhosis and its relation to bacterial infections and prognosis. Hepatology 1984; 4(1):53–8.
17. Deschenes M, Villeneuve J- P. Risk factors for the development of bacterial infections in hospitalized patients with cirrhosis. Am J Gastroenterol 1999;94(8): 2193–7.
18. Saab S, Hernandez JC, Chi AC, et al. Oral antibiotic prophylaxis reduces spontaneous bacterial peritonitis occurrence and improves short-term survival in cirrhosis: a meta-analysis. Am J Gastroenterol 2009;104(4):993–1001.
19. Neill MA, Carpenter CC. Other pathogenic vibrios. In: Mandell GL, Bennett JE, Dolin R, editors. Principles and practice of infectious diseases. 7th edition. Philadelphia: Churchill Livingstone; 2009. p. 2787–90.
20. Daniels Nicholas A, MacKinnon L, Bishop R, et al. Vibrio parahaemolyticus infections in the United States, 1973–1998. J Infect Dis 2000;181(5):1661–6.
21. Balter S, Hanson H, Kornstein L, et al. Vibrio parahaemolyticus infections associated with consumption of raw shellfish—three States, 2006. MMWR Morb Mortal Wkly Rep 2006;55(31):854–6.
22. Dechet Amy M, Yu Patricia A, Koram N, et al. Nonfoodborne Vibrio infections: an important cause of morbidity and mortality in the United States, 1997–2006. Clin Infect Dis 2008;46(7):970–6.
23. Jones MK, Oliver JD. Vibrio vulnificus: disease and pathogenesis. Infect Immun 2009;77(5):1723–33.
24. Klontz KC, Lieb S, Schreiber M, et al. Syndromes of Vibrio vulnificus infections. Ann Intern Med 1988;109(4):318–23.
25. Janda JM, Graves M. Capnocytophaga. In: Mandell GL, Bennett JE, Dolin R, editors. Principles and practice of infectious diseases. 7th edition. Philadelphia: Churchill Livingstone; 2009. p. 2991–4.
26. Brenner DJ, Hollis DG, Fanning GR, et al. Capnocytophaga canimorsus sp. nov. (formerly CDC group DF-2), a cause of septicemia following dog bite, and C. cynodegmi sp. nov., a cause of localized wound infection following dog bite. J Clin Microbiol 1989;27(2):231–5.
27. Janda JM, Graves MH, Lindquist D, et al. Diagnosing Capnocytophaga canimorsus infections. Emerg Infect Dis 2006;12(2):340–2.
28. Deshmukh PM, Camp CJ, Rose FB, et al. Capnocytophaga canimorsus sepsis with purpura fulminans and symmetrical gangrene following a dog bite in a shelter employee. Am J Med Sci 2004;327(6):369–72.
29. Oehler RL, Velez AP, Mizrachi M, et al. Bite-related and septic syndromes caused by cats and dogs. Lancet Infect Dis 2009;9(7):439–47.
30. Bottone EJ. Yersinia enterocolitica: overview and epidemiologic correlates. Microbes Infect 1999;1(4):323–33.
31. Brann OS. Infectious complications of cirrhosis. Curr Gastroenterol Rep 2001; 3(4):285–92.
32. Reed Robert P, Robins-Browne Roy M, Williams Michele L. Yersinia enterocolitica peritonitis. Clin Infect Dis 1997;25(6):1468–9.
33. Guerrant Richard L, Van Gilder T, Steiner Ted S, et al. Practice guidelines for the management of infectious diarrhea. Clin Infect Dis 2001;32(3):331–51.
34. Steinberg JP, Burd EM. Other gram-negative and gram-variable bacilli. In: Mandell GL, Bennett JE, Dolin R, editors, Principles and practice of infectious diseases, vol. 2. Philadelphia: Churchill Livingstone; 2009. p. 3016–9.

35. Ko WC, Lee HC, Chuang YC, et al. Clinical features and therapeutic implications of 104 episodes of monomicrobial *Aeromonas* bacteraemia. J Infect 2000;40(3): 267–73.
36. Llopis F, Grau I, Tubau F, et al. Epidemiological and clinical characteristics of bacteraemia caused by *Aeromonas* spp. as compared with *Escherichia coli* and *Pseudomonas aeruginosa*. Scand J Infect Dis 2004;36(5):335–41.
37. Choi JP, Lee SO, Kwon HH, et al. Clinical significance of spontaneous *Aeromonas* bacterial peritonitis in cirrhotic patients: a matched case-control study. Clin Infect Dis 2008;47(1):66–72.
38. Wu CJ, Lee HC, Chang TT, et al. *Aeromonas* spontaneous bacterial peritonitis: a highly fatal infectious disease in patients with advanced liver cirrhosis. J Formos Med Assoc 2009;108(4):293–300.
39. Jayaraj K, Di Bisceglie AM, Gibson S. Spontaneous bacterial peritonitis caused by infection with *Listeria monocytogenes*: a case report and review of the literature. Am J Gastroenterol 1998;93(9):1556–8.
40. Nolla-Salas J, Almela M, Gasser I, et al. Spontaneous *Listeria monocytogenes* peritonitis: a population-based study of 13 cases collected in Spain. Am J Gastroenterol 2002;97(6):1507–11.
41. Bennett L. Listeria monocytogenes. In: Mandell GL, Bennett JE, Dolin R, editors, Principles and practice of infectious diseases, vol. 2. Philadelphia: Churchill Livingstone; 2009. p. 2707–14.
42. Merle-Melet M, Dossou-Gbete L, Maurer P, et al. Is amoxicillin-cotrimoxazole the most appropriate antibiotic regimen for Listeria meningoencephalitis? Review of 22 cases and the literature. J Infect 1996;33(2):79–85.
43. Soares-Weiser K, Brezis M, Tur-Kaspa R, et al. Antibiotic prophylaxis for cirrhotic patients with gastrointestinal bleeding. Cochrane Database Syst Rev 2002;2:CD002907.
44. Gustot T, Durand F, Lebrec D, et al. Severe sepsis in cirrhosis. Hepatology 2009; 50(6):2022–33.
45. Foreman MG, Mannino DM, Moss M. Cirrhosis as a risk factor for sepsis and death: analysis of the national hospital discharge survey. Chest 2003;124(3): 1016–20.
46. Kumar AM, Roberts DM, Wood KED, et al. Duration of hypotension before initiation of effective antimicrobial therapy is the critical determinant of survival in human septic shock. Crit Care Med 2006;34(6):1589–96.
47. Ibrahim EH, Sherman G, Ward S, et al. The influence of inadequate antimicrobial treatment of bloodstream infections on patient outcomes in the ICU setting. Chest 2000;118(1):146–55.
48. Campillo B, Dypeyron C, Richardet JP. Epidemiology of hospital-acquired infections in cirrhotic patients: effect of carriage of methicillin-resistant *Staphylococcus aureus* and influence of previous antibiotic therapy and norfloxacin prophylaxis. Epidemiol Infect 2001;127(3):443–50.
49. Qurishi N, Kreuzberg C, Luchters G, et al. Effect of antiretroviral therapy on liver-related mortality in patients with HIV and hepatitis C virus coinfection. Lancet 2003;362(9397):1708–13.
50. Loguercio C, Federico A, Tuccillo C, et al. Beneficial effects of a probiotic VSL#3 on parameters of liver dysfunction in chronic liver diseases. J Clin Gastroenterol 2005;39(6):540–3.
51. Stadlbauer V, Mookerjee RP, Hodges S, et al. Effect of probiotic treatment on deranged neutrophil function and cytokine responses in patients with compensated alcoholic cirrhosis. J Hepatol 2008;48(6):945–51.

52. Besselink MGH, van Santvoort HC, Buskens E, et al. Probiotic prophylaxis in pre-dicted severe acute pancreatitis: a randomised, double-blind, placebo-controlled trial. Lancet 2008;371(9613):651–9.
53. Fujita T. Probiotics for patients with liver cirrhosis. J Hepatol 2008;49(6):1080–1.
54. Advisory Committee on Immunization Practices. Recommended adult immuniza-tion schedule: United States, 2010. Ann Intern Med 2010;152(1):36–8.
55. Flechner SM, Avery RK, Fisher R, et al. A randomized prospective controlled trial of oral acyclovir versus oral ganciclovir for cytomegalovirus prophylaxis in high-risk kidney transplant recipients. Transplantation 1998; 66(12):1682–8.
56. Gourishankar S, Wong W, Dorval M. Meta-analysis of prophylaxis of CMV disease in solid organ transplantation: is ganciclovir a superior agent to acyclovir? Trans-plant Proc 2001;33(1–2):1870–2.
57. Winston DJ, Wirin D, Shaked A, et al. Randomised comparison of ganciclovir and high-dose acyclovir for long-term cytomegalovirus prophylaxis in liver-transplant recipients. Lancet 1995;346(8967):69–74.
58. Subramanian A, Dorman S. Mycobacterium tuberculosis in solid organ transplant recipients. Am J Transplant 2009;9(Suppl 4):S57–62.
59. Mazurek GH, Weis SE, Moonan PK, et al. Prospective comparison of the tuber-culin skin test and 2 whole-blood interferon-gamma release assays in persons with suspected tuberculosis. Clin Infect Dis 2007;45(7):837–45.
60. Mazurek GH, Zajdowicz MJ, Hankinson AL, et al. Detection of Mycobacterium tuberculosis infection in United States Navy recruits using the tuberculin skin test or whole-blood interferon-gamma release assays. Clin Infect Dis 2007; 45(7):826–36.
61. Lee SS, Chou KJ, Su IJ, et al. High prevalence of latent tuberculosis infection in patients in end-stage renal disease on hemodialysis: comparison of Quantiferon-TB Gold, Elispot, and tuberculin skin test. Infection 2009;37(2):96–102.
62. Triverio PA, Bridevaux PO, Roux-Lombard P, et al. Interferon-gamma release assays versus tuberculin skin testing for detection of latent tuberculosis in chronic haemodialysis patients. Nephrol Dial Transplant 2009;24(6):1952–6.
63. Manuel O, Humar A, Preiksaitis J, et al. Comparison of quantiferon-TB gold with tuberculin skin test for detecting latent tuberculosis infection prior to liver trans-plantation. Am J Transplant 2007;7(12):2797–801.
64. Ponce de Leon D, Acevedo-Vasquez E, Alvizuri S, et al. Comparison of an interferon-gamma assay with tuberculin skin testing for detection of tuberculosis (TB) infection in patients with rheumatoid arthritis in a TB-endemic population. J Rheumatol 2008;35(5):776–81.
65. Stephan C, Wolf T, Goetsch U, et al. Comparing quantiferon-tuberculosis gold, T-SPOT tuberculosis and tuberculin skin test in HIV-infected individuals from a low prevalence tuberculosis country. AIDS 2008;22(18):2471–9.
66. Takahashi H, Shigehara K, Yamamoto M, et al. Interferon gamma assay for de-tecting latent tuberculosis infection in rheumatoid arthritis patients during inflixi-mab administration. Rheumatol Int 2007;27(12):1143–8.
67. Roland ME, Barin B, Carlson L, et al. HIV-infected liver and kidney transplant recipients: 1- and 3-year outcomes. Am J Transplant 2008;8:355–65.
68. Unos. Center specific report Table 11 summary: 1 year patient survival, adult [PDF]. Available at: http://www.ustransplant.org/csr/current/csrDefault.aspx; 2010. Accessed January 28, 2010.
69. Nakamura N, Tamaru S, Ohshima K, et al. Prognosis of HTLV-1-positive renal transplant recipients. Transplant Proc 2005;37(4):1779–82.

70. Fischer SA, Avery RK. Screening of donor and recipient prior to solid organ trans-plantation. Am J Transplant 2009;9(Suppl 4):S7–18.
71. The National Library of Medicine - National Institute of Health. DailyMed. Available at: http://dailymed.nlm.nih.gov/dailymed/. Accessed March 6, 2010.
72. Panel on Antiretroviral Guidelines for Adults and Adolescents. Guidelines for the use of antiretroviral agents in HIV-1-infected adults and adolescents. Department of Health and Human Services. Available at: http://www.aidsinfo.nih.gov/ContentFiles/AdultandAdolescentGL.pdf; 2009. Accessed March 6, 2010.
73. Wyles David L, Gerber John G. Antiretroviral drug pharmacokinetics in hepatitis with hepatic dysfunction. Clin Infect Dis 2005;40(1):174–81.

Management of Ascites

Preeti A. Reshamwala, MD

KEYWORDS

• Ascites • Portal hypertension • Management
• Serum to ascites albumin gradient • Cirrhosis

Ascites is the abnormal collection of fluid in the peritoneal cavity, and it is the most common complication of cirrhosis.[1] Approximately 85% of all cases of ascites are caused by cirrhosis of the liver. It is also the most common complication of cirrhosis that leads to hospitalization and use of health care resources.[2] During a 10-year observation period, approximately 50% of all cirrhotic patients will develop ascites.[1] The development of ascites heralds a downward medical trajectory for patients with cirrhosis, as 15% die in 1 year, and up to 45% will pass within 5 years.[3] Thus, the management of ascites is critical to quality of life, as well as long-term outcomes both before and after liver transplant.

As noted, most patients with ascites in the United States have cirrhosis, and a new diagnosis of ascites should prompt a careful discussion of the risk factors associated with the development of liver disease. There are several noncirrhotic etiologies of ascites, however, and consideration should be given to these diagnoses when evaluating a patient for the first time presenting with ascites **Box 1**. The physical examination of a patient with presumed ascites often reveals bulging flanks and flank dullness to percussion. Shifting dullness (ie, the change in dullness to percussion that results from shift in free peritoneal fluid on rotation of the patient) is also sensitive for the detection of the presence of ascites.[4] Other stigmata of chronic, advanced liver disease such as jaundice, fetor hepaticus, gynecomastia in males, muscle wasting, spider angioma, and asterixis, also support an underlying diagnosis of cirrhosis. Unfortunately, with the current obesity epidemic, these physical examination findings may be subtle at best, and further diagnostic modalities may be required to confirm the presence of ascites.

The initial interview of a patient with suspected ascites should include a thorough discussion of both current and remote alcohol ingestion, and any past history of drug use. It is estimated that 40 to 80 g of daily alcohol intake over a period of 10 to 20 years is required to develop cirrhosis, although age, gender, and other influences play a role in early development of cirrhosis. Viral hepatitis is commonly acquired via

Digestive Diseases and Transplantation, Emory University School of Medicine, Emory Healthcare, 1365 Clifton Road NE, Building B, Suite 1200, Atlanta, GA 30322, USA
E-mail address: presham@emory.edu

Crit Care Nurs Clin N Am 22 (2010) 309–314
doi:10.1016/j.ccell.2010.04.003   **ccnursing.theclinics.com**

> **Box 1**
> **Etiologies of ascites**
>
> Cirrhosis
>
> Acute hepatitis (eg, alcoholic, viral, autoimmune, drug-induced)
>
> Heart failure
>
> Kidney failure/nephritic syndrome
>
> Cancer/carcinomatosis
>
> Pancreatitis
>
> Sinusoidal obstruction syndrome
>
> Budd Chiari syndrome
>
> Pancreatitis
>
> Mixed
>
> Acute liver failure
>
> Postoperative bile or lymph leak

intravenous drug use, and this history should be thoroughly investigated also. A past history of blood transfusions, travel, tattoos, and needle stick injuries should be queried if viral hepatitis is a concern. A positive family history of liver disease should prompt an investigation for genetic conditions known to be associated with cirrhosis such as alpha one antitrypsin deficiency or Wilson disease. A personal or family history of autoimmune disorders necessitates evaluation for autoimmune hepatitis, primary biliary cirrhosis, or primary sclerosing cholangitis. Obese patients, or those with other risk factors for nonalcoholic fatty liver disease, who have been excluded from having any of the conditions noted, can be evaluated for this condition. A detailed history of cancer, heart failure, kidney disease, and infections also will help determine the potential etiology of ascites. It is important to consider that ascites may be multifactorial, for example, peritonitis in the setting of alcoholic cirrhosis, and therefore appropriate therapy should be aimed at the underlying cause(s). In many patients, the institution of therapy directed to the underling etiology of the ascites often results in an improvement in symptoms.

The diagnosis of ascites can be made reliably with a history and physical examination, as well as a few simple tests. Approximately 1500 cc of fluid must be present to detect flank dullness.[4] An abdominal ultrasound can confirm the presence of free abdominal fluid. Ultrasound is cost-effective, does not expose the patient to radiation, and is easily available at the bedside. It also can be used to mark a site on the abdominal wall that can be used to perform a paracentesis. Other cross-sectional imaging such as triple-phase computed tomography (CT) scan or magnetic resonance imaging (MRI) with and without contrast can be used on a more scheduled basis to evaluate for hepatocellular carcinoma, portal vein thrombosis, splenomegaly, or other signs of portal hypertension.

Once a diagnosis of ascites is established, paracentesis with appropriate testing of the fluid is necessary to understand the etiology of ascites.[5] Evaluation of the serum to ascites albumin gradient (SAAG) can help differentiate portal hypertensive versus nonportal hypertensive causes of ascites.[6] The fluid analysis also can identify the presence of infection, defined as a total white cell count of greater than 250 mm^3 neutrophils. The treatment of peritonitis is critical, as patients can become critically ill with multiorgan failure very quickly.

A bedside paracentesis can be performed rapidly and safely. Complications of paracentesis when using current catheter based equipment trays have been reported to be as low as 1% despite high prevalence of abnormal coagulation parameters.[7] In fact, in a large study looking at bleeding complications from paracentesis, eight of nine patients with reported bleeding after paracentesis had renal failure, suggesting a qualitative platelet abnormality as a contributing etiology of the bleeding. The use of plasma or platelet transfusions, although widely given by practitioners, is not supported by evidence in the literature. In a large study of large volume paracentesis, there were no bleeding complications despite no infusion of preprocedure plasma or platelet transfusions, platelet counts as low as 19,000 cells/mm^3, and international normalized ratio (INR) values as high as 8.7.[8] Although there is no data-supported cutoff at which paracentesis should not be performed, the presence of active bleeding or disseminated intravascular coagulation should preclude performing a paracentesis.

To perform a paracentesis, a site on the lower abdominal wall, preferably the left lower quadrant, should be selected two finger breadths inferior and two finger breadths medial to the anterior superior iliac spine, typically after confirmation with an ultrasound reveals the presence of fluid.[9] The right lower quadrant also can be used as a site for paracentesis; however, there is concern for inadvertent puncture of a dilated cecum, perhaps due to chronic lactulose use. Care should be given in avoiding the inferior epigastric artery and any obvious venous collaterals on the abdominal wall. A midline site halfway between the pubis and umbilicus traditionally had been used in the past; however, concern for bladder puncture and midline collateral vessels, as well as complications of obesity, have steered practitioners away from this site.

Once ascites fluid is obtained, it should be sent to the laboratory to be analyzed for certain basic tests, with secondary testing if differential diagnosis is suggestive of noncirrhotic causes of the ascites (**Table 1**). High cell counts with greater than 250 PMN mm^3 with other features suggestive of spontaneous bacterial peritonitis should prompt inoculation of blood culture bottles with ascites fluid, which can yield a specific bacterium in about 50% of cases.[10] An SAAG is measured by subtracting the albumin value in the ascites fluid from the albumin value in the serum measured on the same day. If the SAAG is greater than 1.1 g/dL, portal hypertension is the cause of ascites, with an accuracy of 97%.[6] Ascitic fluid cytology requires a sample of at least 20 to 50 cc, and should be processed immediately. The sensitivity of cytology in diagnosing peritoneal carcinomatosis is approximately 97% if three fresh samples are submitted and processed quickly.[11] The sensitivity of acid-fast bacilli smear to detect tuberculosis is quite poor, so a culture should be obtained when a high suspicion of tuberculosis peritonitis is suspected. However, a laparoscopic peritoneal biopsy often will be required for definitive testing and diagnosis.

Table 1
Ascites fluid laboratory evaluation

Cell count and differential	Glucose
Albumin	Amylase
Total protein	AFB smear and culture
Culture (preferably in blood culture bottles)	Cytology
Gram's stain	Triglyceride
Lactate dehydrogenase	Bilirubin

Treatment of ascites depends, of course, on the underlying etiology. Those patients with acute alcoholic hepatitis respond dramatically to the cessation of alcohol and nutritional support. Patients with chronic active untreated hepatitis B also can show significant improvement in ascites and synthetic function when started on antiviral agents, with reduction in hepatic necroinflammation.[12] For those patients with portal hypertension and cirrhosis (SAAG >1.1 g/dL), sodium restriction and diuretics are they mainstay of treatment.[13] A 2000 mg/d sodium diet is recommended. Fluid restriction is generally not helpful, and can precipitate volume depletion in an already tenuous patient. If the serum sodium is less than 120 to 125 mmol/L, however, initiation of fluid restriction may be reasonable.

Diuretic regimens traditionally consist of initiating morning doses of furosemide 40 mg/d and spironolactone 100 mg/d. This combination of medications has been shown to reduce time to mobilization of ascites.[14] It also helps to maintain normokalemia, which can be problematic in these patients. Single-agent spironolactone as a starting regimen also is used widely; however, most patients ultimately require the addition of furosemide for maximal efficacy. These medications can be increased every 3to 5 days, while maintaining the ratios, if there is an appropriate weight loss while maintaining renal function. In patients who have massive edema, there is no limit to diuresis and weight loss. Once peripheral edema is resolved, a daily maximum weight loss of no more than 2 kg is recommended. Maximal doses of diuretics that are considered safe for oral intake are 160 mg of furosemide and 400 mg of spironolactone. Single morning doses are recommended to maximize compliance. Painful gynecomastia may occur with spironolactone, and amiloride can be substituted. Other diuretics can be considered, such as metolazone, hydrochlorothiazide, or triamterene. However, none of these medications has been studied as rigorously with data-supported outcomes as furosemide and spironolactone.

For over 90% of patients, the use of diuretics and sodium restriction is effective in achieving reduction in ascites to an acceptable level.[15] In a smaller group of patients, however, these conservative therapies are not sufficient, and large-volume paracentesis may be required. A 5 L paracentesis can be performed safely for the treatment of tense ascites for those patients who are diuretic resistant.[16] For paracenteses of larger volume than 5 L, albumin replacement—8 g/L of fluid removed—has been shown to decrease renal dysfunction and overall morbidity.[17] Unfortunately, refractory ascites occurs when maximal diuretics are being administered, and ascites accumulates rapidly despite paracentesis. Options for managing refractory ascites include serial large volume paracentesis, transjugular intrahepatic portosystemic shunt (TIPS), surgical shunt, and liver transplantation.

Serial large volume paracentesis can be safely performed in patients as frequently as every 10 to 14 days.[5] This, however, can result in a poor quality of life for patients, and consideration for transjugular intrahepatic portosystemic shunts (TIPS) and liver transplantation should be given at this point. TIPS are portocaval shunts that are placed by interventional radiologists. Several large-scale randomized controlled trials have shown superiority of TIPS when compared with serial large volume paracentesis for the control of ascites.[18–20] No significant survival advantage was noted in these studies; however, there was a tendency for more severe hepatic encephalopathy in the TIPS group.[19] TIPS generally should not be placed in patients with severe heart failure, pulmonary hypertension, portal vein thrombosis, advanced hepatocellular carcinoma, and a high Model for End Stage Liver Disease (MELD) score. The development and usage of polytetrafluoroethylene-covered stents have improved longer-term patency for patients, with less of the resultant complications.

Surgical peritoneovenous shunts (LeVeen and Denver) were more commonplace in the 1980s before the advent and widespread use of the more minimally invasive TIPS. However, the end-stage liver patient with refractory ascites is at high risk for any major surgical procedure. Patients with the surgical shunts have a 1-year survival of approximately 60% to 65%, with most patient death occurring in the perioperative period.[21] Additionally, there is low long-term patency of these shunts, with high rates of recurrent portal hypertension, and thus TIPS essentially has obviated the need for these procedures. Surgical shunts should be reserved for those patients who are not candidates for serial paracenteses or TIPS, by a surgeon who has experience in performing these procedures.

Ascites, specifically refractory ascites, is an indication for referral for liver transplantation. As noted previously, the onset of ascites heralds a high 1- and 4-year mortality for patients with end-stage liver disease, so evaluation of candidacy for liver transplantation is warranted. The evaluation process for liver transplantation is extensive, and reviewed elsewhere.[22] Liver transplantation, however, is the definitive treatment of portal hypertension, which is the most common cause of ascites in the United States.

REFERENCES

1. Gines P, Quintero E, Arroyo V, et al. Compensated cirrhosis: natural history and prognostic factors. Hepatology 1987;7(1):122–8.
2. Lucena MI, Andrade RJ, Tognoni G, et al. Multicenter hospital study on prescribing patterns for prophylaxis and treatment of complications of cirrhosis. Eur J Clin Pharmacol 2002;58(6):435–40.
3. Planas R, Montoliu S, Balleste B, et al. Natural history of patients hospitalized for management of cirrhotic ascites. Clin Gastroenterol Hepatol 2006;4(11):1385–94.
4. Cattau EL Jr, Benjamin SB, Knuff TE, et al. The accuracy of the physical examination in the diagnosis of suspected ascites. JAMA 1982;247(8):1164–6.
5. Runyon BA. Care of patients with ascites. N Engl J Med 1994;330(5):337–42.
6. Runyon BA, Montano AA, Akriviadis EA, et al. The serum-ascites albumin gradient is superior to the exudate–transudate concept in the differential diagnosis of ascites. Ann Intern Med 1992;117(3):215–20.
7. Runyon BA. Paracentesis of ascitic fluid. A safe procedure. Arch Intern Med 1986;146(11):2259–61.
8. Grabau CM, Crago SF, Hoff LK, et al. Performance standards for therapeutic abdominal paracentesis. Hepatology 2004;40(2):484–8.
9. Sakai H, Sheer TA, Mendler MH, et al. Choosing the location for non-image guided abdominal paracentesis. Liver Int 2005;25(5):984–6.
10. Runyon BA, Canawati HN, Akriviadis EA. Optimization of ascitic fluid culture technique. Gastroenterology 1988;95(5):1351–5.
11. Runyon BA, Hoefs JC, Morgan TR. Ascitic fluid analysis in malignancy-related ascites. Hepatology 1988;8(5):1104–9.
12. Yao FY, Bass NM. Lamivudine treatment in patients with severely decompensated cirrhosis due to replicating hepatitis B infection. J Hepatol 2000;33(2):301–7.
13. Runyon BA. Management of adult patients with ascites due to cirrhosis: an update. Hepatology 2009;49(6):2087–107.
14. Santos J, Planas R, Pardo A, et al. Spironolactone alone or in combination with furosemide in the treatment of moderate ascites in nonazotemic cirrhosis. A randomized comparative study of efficacy and safety. J Hepatol 2003;39(2):187–92.
15. Stanley MM, Ochi S, Lee KK, et al. Peritoneovenous shunting as compared with medical treatment in patients with alcoholic cirrhosis and massive ascites.

Veterans Administration Cooperative Study on Treatment of Alcoholic Cirrhosis with Ascites. N Engl J Med 1989;321(24):1632–8.

16. Peltekian KM, Wong F, Liu PP, et al. Cardiovascular, renal, and neurohumoral responses to single large-volume paracentesis in patients with cirrhosis and diuretic-resistant ascites. Am J Gastroenterol 1997;92(3):394–9.

17. Tito L, Gines P, Arroyo V, et al. Total paracentesis associated with intravenous albumin management of patients with cirrhosis and ascites. Gastroenterology 1990;98(1):146–51.

18. Rossle M, Ochs A, Gulberg V, et al. A comparison of paracentesis and transjugular intrahepatic portosystemic shunting in patients with ascites. N Engl J Med 2000;342(23):1701–7.

19. Gines P, Uriz J, Calahorra B, et al. Transjugular intrahepatic portosystemic shunting versus paracentesis plus albumin for refractory ascites in cirrhosis. Gastroenterology 2002;123(6):1839–47.

20. Salerno F, Merli M, Riggio O, et al. Randomized controlled study of TIPS versus paracentesis plus albumin in cirrhosis with severe ascites. Hepatology 2004; 40(3):629–35.

21. Hillaire S, Labianca M, Borgonovo G, et al. Peritoneovenous shunting of intractable ascites in patients with cirrhosis: improving results and predictive factors of failure. Surgery 1993;113(4):373–9.

22. Murray KF, Carithers RL Jr. AASLD practice guidelines: evaluation of the patient for liver transplantation. Hepatology 2005;41(6):1407–32.

Correction of Coagulopathy in the Setting of Acute Liver Failure

Amit Mahajan, MD[a], Ishaq Lat, PharmD[b,*]

KEYWORDS

• Acute liver failure • Coagulopathy • Hemorrhage • Bleeding

Multisystem organ failure is common in the setting of acute liver failure (ALF). Although typically not thought of as an organ system, the coagulation system also begins to fail, leading to a host of complications that makes management of critically ill ALF patients difficult.

The liver is essential to the maintenance of hemostasis.[1] Hepatocytes are responsible for the synthesis of most coagulation factors, anticoagulant proteins, and components of the fibrinolytic system. Vitamin K–dependent coagulation proteins (factors II, VII, IX, and X; protein C; protein S; and protein Z) in addition to factors V and XIII, fibrinogen, antithrombin, α_2-plasmin inhibitor, and plasminogen are all synthesized by the liver. Additionally, the liver plays a pivotal role in the regulation of fibrinolysis. Removal of activated clotting and fibrinolytic factors, especially tissue plasminogen activator, is mediated through the hepatic reticuloendothelial system.[2] This delicate balance between coagulation and fibrinolysis is a primary function of the liver. Disturbance of this homeostatic balance secondary to liver failure is typically a multifactorial process. Impairment of coagulation factor synthesis, production of dysfunctional coagulation factors, and increased consumption of coagulation factors are all means by which ALF can upset the balance between coagulation and fibrinolysis, leading to life-threatening coagulopathy and bleeding. The liver's role as a pillar of the coagulation system complicates otherwise routine procedural interventions in critical care.

LABORATORY ASSESSMENT

The initial assessment for ALF reveals dramatically elevated serum aminotransferases, low serum glucose levels, and arterial blood gas studies demonstrating respiratory alkalosis. Laboratory tests typically used for determining metabolic derangements and assessing coagulopathy include the following: platelet count,

[a] Department of Medicine-Section of Pulmonary and Critical Care Medicine, University of Chicago Medical Center, 5841 South, Maryland Avenue, Chicago, IL 60637, USA
[b] Medical Intensive Care Unit, Department of Pharmacy Services, University of Chicago Medical Center, MC 0010, Chicago, IL 60637, USA
* Corresponding author.
E-mail address: Ishaq.lat@uchospitals.edu

Crit Care Nurs Clin N Am 22 (2010) 315–321
doi:10.1016/j.ccell.2010.02.001
0899-5885/10/$ – see front matter © 2010 Elsevier Inc. All rights reserved.

fibrinogen level, prothrombin time (PT), activated partial thromboplastin time (aPTT), thrombin time, and fibrin degradation products/D-dimer assays.[2] The bleeding diathesis stems from decreased levels of the aforementioned vitamin K–dependent factors (factors II, V, VII, IX, and X) resulting in prolonged PT and aPTT. Serial measurements of PT and international normalized ratios (INR) are used to prognosticate liver function and status. Thrombocytopenia (platelet count <150,000/μL) occurs in as many as 70% of ALF patients.[3] The pathogenesis of thrombocytopenia in ALF is unclear.

The consumption of clotting factors and platelets in concert with failure of procoagulant and anticoagulant proteins leads to significant challenges in maintaining hemostasis. Despite the physiologic and laboratory derangements, clinically significant bleeding occurs in less than 5% of patients.[4] The summative point is that an acutely deranged INR is not predictive of bleeding.[5,6]

BLEEDING COMPLICATIONS OF ALF DUE TO COAGULOPATHY

In many cases, bleeding complications in the setting of ALF develop idiopathically. Despite the infrequent and spontaneous nature of clinically significant bleeding events, when bleeding-related complications occur, the outcomes can be devastating.

Gastrointestinal Bleeding

Gastrointestinal (GI) bleeding is a well-documented complication of ALF. A large, prospective, multicenter cohort study found that mechanical ventilation for more than 48 hours and coagulopathy were the only significant risk factors for bleeding in critically ill patients of all types.[7] Patients suffering from ALF are theoretically more prone to GI bleeding due to lack of synthesis and consumption of coagulation factors. Additionally, platelet sequestration further increases the risk for GI bleeding. Massive upper GI bleeding used to be a significant cause of mortality.[8] In a randomized controlled trial, the prophylactic administration of a histamine-2 receptor antagonist (H2RA), cimetidine, was significantly effective in reducing the incidence of GI hemorrhage in patients with hepatic failure.[9] As a result, the American Association for the Study of Liver Diseases officially recommends the use of H2RAs or proton pump inhibitors for prophylaxis against acid-related GI bleeding associated with stress.[10]

Intracranial Hemorrhage

Intracranial hemorrhage in the setting of ALF is typically associated with the use of intracranial pressure (ICP) monitoring. In the absence of an ICP monitor, spontaneous intracranial bleeding is rare (<1%). Recent consensus guidelines recommend that ICP monitoring is especially useful in the decision to exclude patients from emergency liver transplantation.[10,11] According to a survey conducted across medical centers in the United States in the early 1990s, there was an overall prevalence of intracranial bleeding of 20% with the procedure.[12] Correction of coagulopathy before insertion of ICP monitoring devices is recommended to reduce the risk of intracranial hemorrhage.[11]

Spontaneous Hemorrhage

Spontaneous hemorrhage in patients with ALF is commonly associated with significantly low platelet counts. Platelet counts are below 100,000 per cubic centimeter in two-thirds of ALF patients at some point during their clinical course, and platelet function is altered.[13] Patients who develop significant bleeding with platelet levels below approximately 50,000/μL should generally be transfused with platelets provided no contraindication exists.[10,11]

MANAGEMENT OF ALF NECESSITATING INVASIVE INTERVENTIONS

The myriad clinical sequelae associated with ALF pose significant challenges to physicians. Multisystem organ failure is often seen in patients suffering from ALF resulting in altered cardiovascular hemodynamics, renal failure (RF), encephalopathy, pulmonary edema, and coagulopathy. Admission to an ICU is standard for close observation and invasive monitoring. Unfortunately, the treatment of ALF along with intensive monitoring often necessitates the need for invasive interventions, such as central line placement, catheter access for renal replacement therapy, and ICP monitoring. The increased risk of bleeding due to reduced coagulation factor synthesis and thrombocytopenia forces clinicians to judge the benefit of invasive procedures versus the possible risk associated with bleeding complications. The commonly used goal of correction of INR to a value of less than or equal to 1.5 to minimize bleeding risk[10,11] remains untested and lacks scientific basis. Management of coagulopathy in ALF is primarily based on clinical expertise rather than substantial evidence-based data. Yet, most clinicians deem intervention a viable possibility with an INR less than or equal to 1.5 and a platelet count greater than 50,000.[11]

Hemodynamic Monitoring

Evaluation and monitoring of systemic hemodynamics are essential to the treatment of ALF. The primary hemodynamic abnormality in ALF is systemic arterial vasodilation due to reduced precapillary sphincter tone, an abnormality that also occurs in sepsis.[14] Early hemodynamic changes include increased portal pressure, splanchnic sequestration of blood, and decreased central venous return.[15] An essential modality for assessing volume status revolves around the placement of a central venous catheter for central venous pressure monitoring, fluid replacement, and vasopressor administration if necessary.

Insertion of a central venous catheter is performed via the Seldinger technique. This technique involves passing a blunt guide wire through a hollow needle, with subsequent dilation of the desired vessel. The tract created by the dilator is then used to advance the catheter into position. The process of central line insertion can be met with difficulty in patients with large habitus, variant anatomy, and poor vasculature. The risk of arterial cannulation and dilation is one of the many dreaded complications of central line placement. Understandably, arterial cannulation and dilation can be devastating in the setting of coagulopathy associated with ALF. The advent of the portable ultrasound device has led to reduction in rate of complications associated with central line placement. Sulek and colleagues[16] demonstrated approximately a 50% reduction in procedure-related complications with use of portable ultrasound compared with the landmark approach. In patients with ALF, the use of ultrasound guidance is strongly recommended. In common treatment scenarios, such as excessive bleeding or hypotension, emergent central access is necessary for resuscitation and vasopressor administration. During these instances, correction of coagulopathy may not be feasible in a timely manner. Use of ultrasound guidance for central line placement may help clinicians visualize vascular anatomy and ensure cannulation of the appropriate vessel while minimizing complications.

Renal Replacement Therapy Access

Approximately 30% to 75% of patients with fulminant hepatic failure or subacute hepatic failure (encephalopathy within 8 weeks of development of jaundice) develop RF with a greater incidence after acetaminophen poisoning.[17] The cause of acute RF in ALF can stem from nephrotoxic effects of the inciting toxin or from a functional

RF resembling the hepatorenal syndrome of cirrhosis. Although azotemia is common, renal replacement therapy in the setting of ALF is typically used to correct fluid overload, acidosis, and electrolyte abnormalities. Initiation of renal replacement therapy, hemodialysis, or continuous venovenous hemofiltration, requires intravenous access into central vasculature. In the acute setting, temporary access catheters, known as Quinton catheters, are large lumen catheters containing 2 separate tubes; 1 carries blood from the patient to the dialysis machine, and the other returns blood to the circulation. Again, placement of these catheters in the groin, under the collar bone, or in the neck must be done cautiously in the setting of coagulopathy associated with ALF.

ICP Monitoring

Intracranial hypertension accounts for approximately 20% to 25% of deaths and may contribute to residual neurologic impairment after recovery in patients with ALF.[18] Osmotic and hemodynamic abnormalities result in cerebral edema within the fixed cavity of the skull leading to dramatic elevations in ICP. Such elevations in ICP can result in fatal herniation. Prompt recognition of elevated ICP can provide clinicians with direction in therapeutic intervention. Measurements of ICP through invasive monitoring may be of major value in determining which patients (by virtue of uncontrollable ICP) should not undergo transplantation.[19] Additionally, Hanid and colleagues[20] recommend routine monitoring of ICP in patients with ALF, as elevations in ICP to over 60 mm Hg are associated with a poor prognosis. Like any procedure in the setting of coagulopathy, insertion an ICP monitoring device can result in significant bleeding. Studies from Silk and coworkersl[21] suggest that elevations in ICP should be treated promptly because tentorial or cerebellar herniation may occur. Epidural monitors are less hazardous than subdural or parenchymal devices, although their sensitivity is lower.[12] Clinicians are faced with the task of evaluating the risk versus benefit of interventional procedures, such as ICP monitoring, in coagulopathic patients with ALF.

STRATEGIES FOR CORRECTING COAGULOPATHY

There are several treatment modalities for the correction of coagulopathy in the setting of ALF. There are many adverse effects associated with each treatment, making it vital for the treatment team to be familiar with each. An important consideration for correction of coagulopathy is that transfusion of packed red blood cells for the treatment of bleeding and resuscitation lacks the vital individual components for coagulation, making it necessary to replete each coagulation product for effective coagulopathy reversal. Additionally, given the full depletion of coagulation proteins, a multicomponent replacement correction strategy may be necessary rather than relying on just one type of corrective therapy.[10]

Fresh Frozen Plasma

Fresh frozen plasma (FFP) is derived from whole plasma, thus it contains many of the necessary coagulant and anticoagulant proteins contained in normally healthy individuals. The main concern with the administration of FFP is volume overload. Other associated risks include disease transmission, anaphylactoid reactions, alloimmunization, and transfusion-related acute lung injury, although all of these risks are rare. Prophylactic administration of FFP to correct the laboratory markers of PT and INR is not recommended because this has never been shown to prevent clinically significant bleeding and obscures the prognosis.[10]

Plasmapharesis

As a therapeutic modality to filter out harmful chemicals and replete necessary proteins, plasmapharesis is an attractive option. Plasmapharesis for the management of ALF has been studied as a therapeutic option to correct coagulopathy.[22] Definitive recommendations regarding its efficacy and wider application are not feasible, however, given the limited sample sizes for study and due to the greater application of liver transplantation. The role of plasmapharesis and its timing in the treatment algorithm remains unclear.

Cryoprecipitate

Cryoprecipitate is derived from human plasma and is stocked in the blood bank at most institutions. Each 15 mL of cryoprecipitate contains 100 IU of factor VIII and 250 mg of fibrinogen.[23] ALF is associated with a dramatic decrease in serum fibrinogen concentrations (serum <100 mg/dL, normal 180–409 mg/dL). In conjunction with the innate depletion of vital coagulant factors, the corresponding reduction in fibrinogen impairs the hosts' ability to clot and to prevent further bleeding. Therefore, it is recommended that for the correction of coagulopathy in ALF cryoprecipitate be administered.

Recombinant Factor VIIa

In recent years, the administration of recombinant factor VIIa has become en vogue. Factor VIIa is an endogenous factor derived from vitamin K and synthesized by the liver. Recombinant factor VIIa (NovoSeven) complexes with tissue factor at the site of injury and this activates coagulation factor X to factor Xa and factor IX to factor IXa. Factor Xa can complex with other factors to aid in the conversion of prothrombin to thrombin, which ultimately generates a hemostatic plug by converting fibrinogen to fibrin, ultimately inducing local hemostasis. The administration of recombinant factor VIIa has several advantages, some of which include: small volume perhaps leading to less volume overload and a rapid correction of laboratory parameters. There are several limitations, however, and adverse effects to be mindful of: the correction of laboratory parameters may not fully reflect hemostasis given the drug's extrinsic affect on the INR test; recombinant factor VIIa is associated with reports of venous and arterial thromboembolism; there is a lack of well-done controlled trials demonstrating its effectiveness; and it has a high cost. Due to the lack of well-controlled research, the lowest effective dose remains to be determined. Additionally, because recombinant factor VIIa is used as a prophylactic therapy to prevent further bleeding, it remains unclear whether or not recombinant factor VIIa is more effective than placebo at preventing bleeding episodes in the setting of ALF. Despite all these limitations, recombinant factor VIIa is recommended for administration before invasive procedures with a high risk of bleeding (ie, transjugular liver biopsy or the placement of an ICP monitor).[10] Recombinant factor VIIa should not be administered to patients with a recent history of thrombosis, myocardial infarction, or ischemic stroke.

SUMMARY

The depletion of vital coagulation factors and proteins in the setting of ALF is common and multifactorial. The management of critically ill patients with ALF is, therefore, difficult and requires a multidisciplinary approach to effective treatment. Critical care nurses are essential in identifying potential sources of bleeding, monitoring for transfusion reactions, and staying vigilant for medication-related adverse reactions. Prevention and treatment of bleeding disorders is a priority because ineffective therapy can lead to hazardous consequences. Correction of coagulopathy for treatment of bleeding and reversal for invasive procedures should include a multifactorial therapeutic plan emphasizing the correction of all coagulation factors. The limitations of current knowledge in effective correction should serve as a stimulus for future research.

REFERENCES

1. Ghany M, Hoofnagle JH. Approach to the patient with liver disease. In: Kasper DL, Braunwald E, Fauci AS, et al, editors. Harrison's principles of internal medicine, vol. 1. 16th edition. New York: McGraw-Hill Companies; 2005. p. 1808–13.
2. Greenberg DL, Davie EW. Blood coagulation factors: their complementary DNAs, genes, and expression. In: Coleman RW, Hirsh J, Marder VJ, et al, editors, Hemostsis & thrombosis: basic principles and clinical practice. 4th edition. Philadelphia: Lippincott, Williams & Wilkins; 2001. p. 21–7.
3. Schiodt FV, Balko J, Schilsky M, et al. Thrombopoietin in acute liver failure. Hepatology 2003;37:558–61.
4. Pereira LM, Langley PG, Hayllar KM, et al. Coagulation factor V and VIII/V ratio as predictors of outcome in paracetamol induced fulminant hepatic failure: relation to other prognostic indicators. Gut 1992;33:98–102.
5. Hugenholt GC, Porte RJ, Lisman T. The platelet and platelet function testing in liver disease. Clin Liver Dis 2009;13:11–20.
6. Lisman T, Leebeek FW. Hemostatic alterations in liver disease: a review on pathophysiology, clinical consequences, and treatment. Dig Surg 2007;24:250–8.
7. Cook DJ, Fuller HD, Guyatt GH, et al. Risk factors for gastrointestinal bleeding in critically ill patients. N Engl J Med 1994;330:377–81.
8. Bailey R, MacDougall B, Williams R. A controlled trial of the H2-receptor antagonists in prophylaxis of bleeding from gastrointestinal tract erosions in fulminant hepatic failure. Gut 1976;17:389.
9. MacDougall B, Bailey R, Williams R. H2-Receptor antagonists and antacids in the presentation of acute upper gastrointestinal haemorrhage in fulminant hepatic failure. Lancet 1977;1:617–9.
10. Polson J, Lee WM. AASLD position paper: the management of acute liver failure. Hepatology 2005;41:1179–97.
11. Stravitz RT, Kramer AH, Davern T. Intensive care of patients with acute liver failure: recommendations of the U.S. Acute Liver Failure Study Group. Crit Care Med 2007;35:2498–508.
12. Blei AT, Olafsson S, Webster S, et al. Complications of intracranial pressure monitoring in fulminant hepatic failure. Lancet 1993;341:157–8.
13. O'Grady JG, Langley PG, Isola LM, et al. Coagulopathy of fulminant hepatic failure. Semin Liver Dis 1986;6:159–63.
14. Guimond J, Pinsky M, Matuschak G. Effect of synchronous increase in intrathoracic pressure on cardiac performance during acute endotoxemia. J Appl Phys 1990;69:1502–8.
15. Pinsky MR, Matuschak G, Bernardi L, et al. Effects of cardiac cycle-specific increases in intrathoracic pressure. J Appl Phys 1986;60:604–12.
16. Sulek CA, Blas ML, Lobato EB. A randomized study of left versus right internal jugular vein cannulation in adults. J Clin Anesth 2000;12:142–5.
17. O'Grady JG, Gimson AE, O'Brien CJ, et al. Controlled trials of charcoal hemoperfusion and prognostic factors in fulminant hepatic failure. Gastroenterology 1988; 94:1186–92.

18. Jackson EW, Zacks S, Zinn S, et al. Delayed neuropsychologic dysfunction after liver transplantation for acute liver failure: a matched, case-controlled study. Liver Transpl 2002;8:932–6.

19. Donovan JP, Shaw BW Jr, Langnas AN, et al. Brain water and acute liver failure: the emerging role of intracranial pressure monitoring. Hepatology 1992;16:267–8.

20. Hanid M, Davies M, Mellon PJ, et al. Clinical monitoring of intracranial pressure in fulminant hepatic failure. Gut 1980;21:866–9.

21. Silk DB, Trewby PN, Chase RA, et al. Treatment of fulminant hepatic failure by polyacrylonitrile-membrane haemodialysis. Lancet 1977;2:1–3.

22. Munoz SJ, Ballas SK, Moritz MJ, et al. Perioperative management of fulminant and subfulminant hepatic failure with therapeutic plasmapharesis. Transplant Proc 1989;21:3535–6.

23. Erber WN, Perry DJ. Plasma and plasma products in the treatment of massive haemorrhage. Best Pract Res Clin Haematol 2006;19:97–112.

Drug-Induced Liver Disease

Jiwon W. Kim, PharmD, BCPS, FCSHP[a],*, Akiko Hattori, PharmD[b],
Paula V. Phongsamran, PharmD[a]

KEYWORDS

- Drug-induced liver disease • Liver injury
- Hepatotoxicity • Drugs

The liver is the major organ responsible for detoxification of various substances, including drugs and toxins. The central role it plays in drug metabolism and clearance makes the liver highly susceptible to drug-induced injury, which accounts for up to 10% of all adverse drug events.[1] Drug-induced liver disease is the leading cause of acute liver failure in the United States and the most common reason for a drug to be withdrawn from the market.[2] More than 1000 drugs have been implicated in causing liver disease. The types of injury to the liver can vary, from minor insults with subclinical liver enzyme abnormalities that resolve upon discontinuation of the offending drug, to fulminant hepatic necrosis.[3] There is no effective treatment for drug-induced liver injury in most cases other than discontinuing the drug and providing general supportive care. Identification and prevention of drug-induced liver disease are the only proven strategies for improving patient outcomes. For health care professionals on the frontline of patient care, better understanding of drug-induced liver injury is vital in avoiding potential adverse drug events and ensuring the best clinical outcomes.

EPIDEMIOLOGY

The reported incidence of drug-induced liver disease is low, ranging from 1 case in 10,000 to 100,000 persons exposed to offending drugs,[4] although the true incidence is difficult to assess because of underreporting and difficulties in the diagnosis of hepatotoxicity.[1] A recently published population-based, case control study, for example, suggests a much higher incidence of drug-induced liver disease, of up to almost 14 cases per 100,000 patients per year.[5] The documentation of the

[a] Department of Clinical Pharmacy and Pharmaceutical Economics and Policy, University of Southern California School of Pharmacy, USC University Hospital, 1500 San Pablo Street, Los Angeles, CA 90033, USA
[b] University of Southern California University Hospital, 1500 San Pablo Street, Los Angeles, CA 90033, USA
* Corresponding author.
E-mail address: jiwonkim@usc.edu

Crit Care Nurs Clin N Am 22 (2010) 323–334
doi:10.1016/j.ccell.2010.02.002 ccnursing.theclinics.com
0899-5885/10/$ – see front matter © 2010 Elsevier Inc. All rights reserved.

epidemiology on drug-induced liver disease is generally poor because of difficulties in diagnosis of the liver injury, relatively low number of epidemiologic studies, and a wide variability in rate of drug-induced liver injury from one drug to another. Available information of causative drugs comes from single case reports, and many cases remain unreported. Reported data estimate that only 1 in 20 drug-induced liver injury cases are reported.[5] The overall incidence of drug-induced liver disease is increasing because of a rising number of new therapeutic agents introduced over the past several decades and higher reporting rates. Data on drug-induced liver disease from the national European registry reported a near doubling of reported cases from 1968 to 1978 to the following decade, 1978 to 1987.[6]

Drug-induced liver disease accounts for about 50% of those who present with acute hepatitis and 10% of consultations by hepatologists.[5,7,8] About 1% of all general medical admissions are related to drug-induced liver injury, which is responsible for 15% of all liver transplantations in the United States.[8] The drugs most responsible for liver injuries are acetaminophen, antimicrobials, psychotropic agents, lipid-lowering agents, and nonsteroidal anti-inflammatory drugs (NSAIDs).

RISK FACTORS

In patients receiving drugs associated with liver injury, recognizing the risk factors for hepatotoxicity is an important strategy to prevent potentially severe drug reactions. Risk factors involved in drug-induced liver disease are multifaceted (**Table 1**). The most common risk factors are advanced age, sex, alcohol use history, pregnancy, and genetic predisposition.[9] Adults are generally more susceptible to liver damage than are children, possibly because of a higher rate of drug use and age-associated impairment in drug disposition and metabolism. Older age, for example, is a known risk factor for liver toxicity associated with isoniazid. Higher prevalence of valproate-induced liver injury, however, has been reported more in children compared with adults.[10] Early reports have suggested that women are more likely to experience liver injury from drugs, especially from methyldopa and diclofenac.[1,11] Men, however, are more prone to hepatotoxicity from drugs such as azathioprine and amoxicillin/clavulanate.[9] Chronic alcohol abuse is an established risk factor for acetaminophen-associated liver injury, with the greatest risk during the period of temporary abstinence from alcohol.[12] Intravenous tetracycline-associated hepatitis has been reported mostly in pregnant women.[9] There are genetic predispositions known to alter metabolism of drugs within the liver. These defects can cause delayed drug metabolism or accumulation of toxic metabolites, resulting in injury.[9] Genetic deficiency in

Table 1 Risk factors for drug-induced liver disease	
Drugs	**Risk Factors**
Acetaminophen	Chronic alcohol abuse, pregnancy, fasting
Diclofenac	Female gender, osteoarthritis
Isoniazid	Chronic alcohol abuse, advanced age, female gender, pregnancy
Methotrexate	Chronic alcohol abuse, chronic liver disease, obesity, diabetes
Phenytoin	Genetic predisposition
Sulfonamide	Female gender, human immunodeficiency virus (HIV) infection, genetic predisposition
Valproic acid	Young age, genetic predisposition

detoxification capacity has been reported for phenytoin, carbamazepine, and sulfon-amides. Chronic liver disease does not appear to increase the risk of drug-induced liver injury, except for drugs such as methotrexate and niacin, which should be avoided in patients with cirrhosis.

PATHOGENESIS

Drug metabolism occurs mainly in the liver, and most drug-associated liver injuries result from the active metabolites of drug biotransformation. Drug metabolism in the liver begins with the phase 1 oxidative pathway, in which the drug undergoes biotrans-formation to a more polar substance mediated by the cytochrome P450 (CYP450) enzyme system. This process is followed by phase 2 reaction, in which the conversion of metabolites forms highly polar sulfates and glucuronides, which generally are excreted renally. Although several other drug metabolism and clearance pathways exist, the primary metabolic pathways for most drugs involve CYP450 and subsequent glucuronidation. Hepatocelluar necrosis occurs when drug metabolites formed by CYP450 activation bind to cellular membranes or DNA and disrupt cell function.[13] The active metabolites also may produce free radicals that can bind to proteins and cause structural or functional lesions. This may either prompt an immune response or damage the cell directly, resulting in cell death, which begins the cascade of the symptoms that characterize hepatitis. Active metabolites of drug biotransformation also can induce liver damage by covalently binding to the liver enzymes, resulting in immune-mediated hepatotoxicity.[13]

CYP450 enzyme system consists of more than 30 different enzymes with interindi-vidual variations in activity and in capacity to be induced or inhibited by other substances. This results in clinically significant drug interactions and increases risk of drug-induced liver injury. CYP450 enzyme polymorphisms may place susceptible individuals at greater risk of drug-induced liver toxicity. In general, those who experi-ence liver injury produce a greater concentration of hepatotoxins from drug metabo-lism. This may be because of genetic deficiencies in liver enzymes necessary for the metabolism and clearance of offending drugs that are associated with liver injury.

Phase 2 reaction of drug metabolism involves the binding of glutathione, glucuro-nate, and sulfate to reactive metabolites and forming nontoxic substances that are readily excreted through bile or urine. Glutathione conjugation protects cellular enzymes and membranes from toxic metabolites and therefore is one of the most important defense mechanisms against hepatocellular injury. Inadequate stores of glutathione can compromise efficient detoxification of the reactive metabolites and can result in liver injury. The rate-limiting factor in glutathione synthesis is the intracel-lular concentration of cysteine, which often is supplied in the form of N-acetylcysteine, which replenishes glutathione in acute acetaminophen toxicity. Other proposed mechanisms of drug-induced liver injury include sensitization of the liver cells to cyto-kines, autoimmune bile duct injury, mitochondrial disruption, and disruption of trans-port proteins.[14]

CLASSIFICATION OF DRUG-INDUCED HEPATOTOXICITY

Hepatotoxicity from drugs is classified into two categories: intrinsic or idiosyncratic. In intrinsic hepatotoxicity, the adverse hepatic event is highly predictable and dose-dependent. Injuries to the liver occur when a toxic amount of drug is consumed. Hepatic injuries present after a short duration of drug ingestion, and this type of hepa-totoxicity usually is identified during drug development within the context of the preclinical animal studies. Acetaminophen, isoniazid, and tetracycline are example of drugs with dose-dependent hepatotoxic effects when higher-than-recommended dosages can cause severe liver injuries (**Table 2**). The drug with the most frequent cases of intrinsic hepatotoxicity is acetaminophen, which can cause extensive hepatic necrosis with as little as 10 to 15 g.[15] Most drug-induced hepatic injuries are unpredictable or idiosyncratic, in which the occurrence is infrequent and may or may not be dose-dependent (**Table 3**). In these cases, there is a variable latency period, and cases are often fatal if the drug continues to be administered once the injury has occurred.[2] Idiosyncratic hepatotoxicity can be classified as allergic or nonallergic, and only a small percentage of individuals exposed to the causative drug experience the liver damage. Idiosyncratic allergic hepatotoxicity may be attributed to hypersensitivity when the presenting symptoms are accompanied by fever, rash, and eosinophilia. The injury usually develops after a sensitization period of 1 to 5 weeks, whereas the injuries seen with nonallergic hepatotoxicity appear after a widely variable latency period. The classic features of hypersensitivity are absent in nonallergic idiosyncratic reactions, and the liver injury may occur weeks to months after drug administration.

CLINICAL SPECTRUM OF DRUG-INDUCED LIVER DISEASE

Drug-induced liver disease manifests itself in several different clinical features depending on the type of drug and the corresponding adverse effect on the liver (**Table 4**). Presenting clinical findings are highly variable, ranging from asymptomatic elevations in liver enzymes to fatal hepatic failure. Most drugs have a unique pattern of hepatotoxicity in time of onset, frequency, and type of hepatic injury. Acute hepatitis is the most common form of clinically significant liver injury, which consists of acute hepatocellular hepatitis, acute cholestatic hepatitis, and mixed-pattern acute hepatitis. Chronic hepatitis, including cirrhosis of the liver, is much less common and often resembles chronic liver disease from other etiologies, such as viral hepatitis and autoimmune hepatitis.

Acute Hepatocellular Hepatitis

Acute hepatocellular hepatitis is the most common drug-induced liver injury, representing up to 90% of the cases, and it can result from a wide variety of drugs.[3,16] Toxic necrosis is acute hepatocellular injury whereby the drug or its metabolite causes direct damage to the cells of the liver. It has a highly predictable occurrence with dose-related hepatotoxicity. The most important example of toxic necrosis is acetaminophen. Most of the drug is metabolized into benign conjugates, which are excreted in urine and bile. Approximately 5% to 9% of acetaminophen is metabolized to the

Table 2	
Drugs with dose-dependent hepatotoxicity	
Drugs	**Hepatotoxicity**
Acetaminophen	Hepatocellular necrosis
Amiodarone	Chronic steatosis
Cyclosporine	Cholestasis
Methotrexate	Fibrosis
Niacin	Vascular injury
Oral contraceptives	Hepatic tumor
Tetracycline	Steatosis

Table 3
Drugs with idiosyncratic liver injuries

Drugs	Forms of Liver Injuries
Isoniazid, trazodone, diclofenac, venlafaxine, lovastatin, telithromycin	Hepatocellular necrosis
Chlorpromazine, estrogen, erythromycin, and other macrolides	Cholestasis
Phenytoin, sulfamethoxazole	Hypersensitivity reaction
Diltiazem, sulfonamides, quinidine	Granulomatous hepatitis
Didanosine, tetracycline, valproic acid	Acute steatosis
Nitrofurantoin, methyldopa, lovastatin, minocycline	Autoimmune hepatitis
Methotrexate	Fibrosis
Amoxicillin/clavulanate, carbamazepine, cyclosporine, methimazole	Mixed hepatocellular/cholestatic injury

toxic metabolite N-acetyl-p-benzoquinone imine, which is metabolized rapidly and conjugated with glutathione, forming a nontoxic substance that is excreted renally. When a significantly large dose of acetaminophen is consumed, the stores of glutathione in the liver are depleted, and the toxic metabolites bind to components of the cells, resulting in hepatic necrosis. Toxic necrosis of the hepatocytes is characterized by marked elevations in alanine aminotransferase (ALT) and aspartate aminotransferase (AST) with variable elevations in bilirubin. Alkaline phosphatase (ALK) value remains normal or only slightly elevated. These biochemical patterns resemble those of acute viral hepatitis, with the exception of immense elevations in liver enzymes without an upper limit, which is common with most drug-induced toxic necrosis but

Table 4
Clinical spectrum of drug-induced liver disease and associated drugs

Type of Liver Injury	Drugs
Toxic necrosis	Acetaminophen, sulfonamides, ketoconazole, isoniazid, rifampin, phenytoin, valproic acid, carbamazepine, diclofenac, labetalol, disulfiram
Acute hepatitis	Methyldopa, nevirapine, ritonavir, minocycline
Cholestasis	Oral contraceptives, anabolic steroids, warfarin
Mixed-pattern hepatocellular/ cholestasis	Macrolide antibiotics, chlorpromazine, azathioprine, amitriptyline, nitrofurantoin, phenytoin, phenobarbital, sulfonamides, verapamil
Chronic hepatitis	Minocycline, nitrofurantoin, fenofibrate, methyldopa, phenytoin, propylthiouracil, diclofenac
Hepatic vein thrombosis	Dacarbazine, oral contraceptives
Veno-occlusive disease	Azathioprine, mercaptopurine, cyclophosphamide, oral contraceptives, tetracycline, pyrrolizidine alkaloids
Steatosis	Corticosteroids, nitrofurantoin, methotrexate, tamoxifen, valproic acid, zidovudine, amiodarone, diltiazem, verapamil
Granulomatous hepatitis	Allopurinol, amiodarone, carbamazepine, diltiazem, isoniazid, methyldopa, phenytoin, quinidine, sulfonamides

unusual with other causes of liver disease. Although many patients who experience hepatocellular necrosis may be asymptomatic, the prognosis is considerably worse if jaundice is present, with mortality rates of 10% or greater.[9] Other clinical features include fatigue, anorexia, and nausea. In patients with fulminant liver failure from hepatocellular necrosis, jaundice, coagulopathy, ascites, hepatic encephalopathy, coma, and death can occur. Other drugs reported to cause hepatocellular necrosis include methyldopa, telithromycin, valproic acid, trazodone, venlafaxine, and lovastatin.[9]

Acute Cholestatic Hepatitis

Acute cholestatic hepatitis is another major clinical presentation in patients with drug-induced liver injury. Cholestasis is a condition in which reduced secretion or obstruction of the biliary tree results in a reduction of bile flow. Acute cholestatic hepatitis is defined as a marked increase in serum ALK concentrations greater than two times the upper limit of normal (ULN) and is characterized mainly by jaundice, pruritus, pale stool, and dark urine. Conjugated bilirubin and γ-glutamyl transpeptidase (GGT) concentrations also are elevated, along with other indicators of bile duct injury. Other presenting features of the cholestatic injury may include abdominal pain, fever, and chills that mimic acute biliary obstruction. In most cases of drug-induced cholestatic hepatitis, symptoms subside once the offending drug is withdrawn, and the prognosis is much better compared with acute hepatocellular hepatitis. Complete recovery may be delayed compared with hepatocellular hepatitis, but typically occurs within a few weeks after the discontinuation of the causative agent. It usually has a good prognosis, with jaundice resolving within a several months. Amoxicillin/clavulanate is one of the most frequent causes of acute cholestatic injury.[17] Other drugs associated with acute cholestasis include chlorpromazine, anabolic steroids, and oral contraceptives.

Mixed-Pattern Acute Hepatitis

Drug-induced injury presenting as a mixed form acute hepatitis can be either primarily hepatocellular with cholestatic features or primarily cholestatic with characteristics of hepatocellular necrosis. Mixed-pattern acute hepatitis is defined as ALT:ALK ratio between 2 and 5 with AST and ALT concentrations elevated to more than eight times the ULN. Jaundice and clinical features resembling cholestasis are commonly present, with the exception of pain and fever, which are much less common with drug-induced mixed injury. The prognosis is usually good, and fulminant hepatitis rarely is seen with mixed injury. Drugs most commonly associated with mixed-pattern injury include tricyclic antidepressants, NSAIDs, macrolides, nitrofurantoin, sulfonamides, amoxicillin/clavulanate, cyclosporine, methimazole, and carbamazepine.[9]

Chronic Hepatitis

Although drug-induced liver injury for the most part is an acute event, some drug-induced hepatotoxicity is associated with an insidious effect that develops into chronic liver disease. Chronic hepatitis caused by drugs is defined by evidence of ongoing hepatic injury for 6 months or longer. It may result from drugs that initially induce acute hepatitis, but which then progress to chronic inflammation with continued use of the offending agent. Chronic hepatitis may be indistinguishable from autoimmune hepatitis, both in clinical symptoms and histologic features. Drug-induced chronic hepatitis typically occurs after a prolonged duration of drug therapy, from several months to years, and the extent of the injury may correlate with the duration of drug use. Most cases of drug-induced chronic hepatitis occur in women, who may experience increase in serum globulin concentrations and presence of serum antinuclear antibodies.[9,18] The clinical onset of chronic hepatitis is variable and may be acute or progress insidiously. Presenting symptoms are similar to those of acute and chronic liver disease, including enlarged liver, splenomegaly, and ascites. Other classic symptoms such as jaundice, anorexia, and fatigue also may be present. Biomarkers of liver injury are elevated aminotransferase concentrations and elevated coagulation markers such as prothrombin time. Withdrawal of the causative drugs usually results in improvement or resolution of the disease within weeks, whereas continued use of the drug may lead to hepatic fibrosis, fulminant liver failure, and death. Drugs associated with drug-induced chronic hepatitis include dantrolene, diclofenac, methyldopa, minocycline, nitrofurantoin, and sulfonamides. Drugs such as acetaminophen, aspirin, and dantrolene produce chronic hepatitis through toxic effects of the drugs, rather than the chronic inflammation of the hepatocytes.

Continued injury to the liver eventually leads to scarring of the affected tissues with subsequent cirrhosis. Clinical manifestations from a drug-induced cause remain typical of those cases of cirrhosis from other causes. Development of cirrhosis may occur through various hepatic injuries, from chronic hepatitis to lesions from chronic intrahepatic cholestasis. In some cases, gradual progression to cirrhosis may be undetectable, as with drugs such as methotrexate, which has increased risk of developing cirrhosis with concomitant use of alcohol and other hepatotoxins.[9] Other associated factors that may increase the risk of methotrexate-associated fibrosis leading to cirrhosis include obesity and diabetes mellitus. Current guidelines for patients taking methotrexate recommend routine monitoring of aminotransferase and albumin concentrations.

Other Forms of Drug-induced Liver Injuries

Other types of drug-induced liver injury include chronic steatosis, vascular injury, granulomatous hepatitis, and neoplastic lesions. Chronic steatosis, a liver disease in which hepatocytes are filled with large vacuoles of fat, has a minimal number of clinical manifestations with the exception of enlarged liver. This often results from prolonged use of the offending drugs such as glucocorticoids, methotrexate, amiodarone, and tamoxifen. Some chronic steatosis is benign, whereas methotrexate-induced steatosis can progress to cirrhosis. Valproic acid has been associated with fatty degeneration that can result in chronic liver failure and severe hepatic necrosis.[9]

Drug-induced hepatic vascular disease is rare but may manifest in several different clinical features. Hepatic vein thrombosis, also referred to as Budd-Chiari syndrome, causes obstruction of the hepatic venous outflow resulting in patients experiencing abdominal pain, ascites, and hepatomegaly. Although rare, hepatic venous thrombosis has been associated with oral contraceptives.[19] Veno-occlusive disease is one of the more serious drug-induced vascular injuries, and it presents as rapid weight gain, ascites, jaundice, and symptoms of portal hypertension. Symptoms may vary from mild hepatitis to fatal hepatic failure. Veno-occlusive disease associated with drugs may have an abrupt onset of clinical symptoms from a large amount of drug ingestion or it may have an insidious onset from exposure to small dosages of causative drugs for a prolonged period. The acute form of injury is generally reversible, but may be fatal. Drugs associated with veno-occlusive disease include azathioprine, mercaptopurine, and cyclophosphamide, along with oral contraceptives, tetracycline, and plant alkaloids found in dietary supplements.[9]

Drug-induced granulomatous hepatitis is usually characterized by the presence of fever, diaphoresis, malaise, anorexia, jaundice, or right upper quadrant discomfort. A granuloma, which is a presence of clusters of inflammatory cells within the liver, usually results from the immune-mediated response to the causative agents.

Symptoms usually occur between 10 days and 4 months after the initiation of drug therapy, with splenomegaly presenting in up 15% of cases. Several drugs, including amiodarone, allopurinol, and carbamazepine, have been implicated in drug-induced granulomatous hepatitis; up to 60 drugs have been associated with hepatic granulomas.

There have been numerous reports of drugs linked to neoplasms of the liver, both benign and malignant forms. The use of oral contraceptives and anabolic steroids has been linked to hepatic adenoma, which is a benign tumor of the liver. Hepatocellular carcinoma and adenoma have been described in women with history of oral contraceptive use, with relative risk of more than 100-fold in those exposed to the drugs for more than 10 years.[20] The most recent meta-analysis, however, suggests a lack of association between oral contraceptives and liver cancer, possibly because of the rare incidence of liver tumors.[21]

Dietary Supplement-induced Liver Disease

As dietary supplements are widely used with continuing popularity, an increasing number of liver injuries caused by dietary supplements have been reported. Hepatotoxicity from dietary supplements ranges from mild and self-limiting symptoms to life-threatening conditions such as liver failure. Most recently, the popular weight-loss product Hydroxycut was removed from the market because of several serious hepatotoxicities. The spectrum of dietary supplement-induced liver disease encompasses all forms of liver injuries, including minor elevations in liver enzymes, acute and chronic hepatitis, steatosis, cholestasis, hepatocellular necrosis, hepatic fibrosis, veno-occlusive disease, and acute liver failure.[22] Dietary supplements are not subject to rigorous testing or regulation, and a standard manufacturing process does not exist. Consequently, safety information on these products is not readily available, and potential hepatotoxicity risk is not known until multiple cases are reported.

The hepatotoxic effects of comfrey are caused by pyrrolizidine alkaloids, which have been associated with veno-occlusive disease, with a mortality rate of up to 40% in cases of acute liver failure.[23] Jin bu Huan is commonly used as a sedative and analgesic but is associated with at least 10 cases of acute hepatitis, which appears to be an immune-mediated drug reaction.[24] Presenting symptoms reported are fever, fatigue, nausea, pruritus, abdominal pain, jaundice, and hepatomegaly. Several cases of kava-associated hepatotoxicity, including one with hepatic failure requiring liver transplantation, have been reported.[25] Other dietary supplements implicated in liver injury include chaparral leaf, camphor, gentian, germander, and valerian.[26]

Green tea contains catechin polyphenols, known to possess antioxidant, anticarcinogenic, and antitumorigenic properties. Green tea extracts are widely available and are commonly used as a key ingredient in several dietary supplements for varying uses. There have been a growing number of cases of liver injury associated with green tea extract.[27] *Camellia senesis* is the major ingredient of green tea extract supplements and most likely is the hepatotoxin responsible for the liver injury. The presenting symptoms of liver toxicity associated with green tea extract are portal inflammation and cholestasis after 5 days of use. Markedly elevated aminotransferase concentrations and hepatocellular necrosis after 5 weeks of use also have been reported with green tea extract. Upon prompt discontinuation of the supplement, complete resolution of the symptoms generally has been observed, although several cases of acute liver failure requiring liver transplantation have been reported.

MANAGEMENT OF DRUG-INDUCED LIVER DISEASE

The first step in managing patients with drug-induced liver injury is to correctly identify and withdraw the offending agent and give an antidote, if available. N-acetylcysteine is the established antidote for acetaminophen toxicity caused by an acute overdose. The mechanism of action is the replenishment of glutathione stores. The most widely practiced management of acute single-time point overdose is the Rumack-Matthew nomogram, which provides guidance in determining the risk of hepatotoxicity.[28] Serum acetaminophen concentrations measured 4 hours after and within 24 hours of drug ingestion can be used with the nomogram to assess the level of risk for developing hepatotoxicity. This information then can be used to determine whether N-acetylcysteine can be used successfully to treat acetaminophen-induced hepatic necrosis and prevent liver failure. Both the oral and intravenous formulations of N-acetylcysteine appear to be equally efficacious in treating acetaminophen-induced hepatotoxicity.[29–31] The oral formulation of N-acetylcysteine has a minimal adverse effect profile, consisting mostly of nausea and vomiting. The intravenous formulation of N-acetylcysteine, used infrequently because of the cost and the risk of anaphylaxis, has several adverse effects including pruritus, flushing, and rash. Although bronchospasm and hypotension occur rarely, fatal reactions have been reported with the use of intravenous N-acetylcysteine.

Other drug-induced liver diseases have no specific treatment other than providing supportive care, since most cases resolve spontaneously. In these cases, identifying and discontinuing the administration of the offending agent are the most important steps in preventing the injury from progressing to fatal liver failure. Early referral for liver transplantation is essential for patient survival for those with predictive variables of death, such as age greater than 65 years, bilirubin 18 times the ULN, AST greater than 34 times the ULN, ALT greater than 31 times the ULN, and prothrombin time greater than 100 seconds. Corticosteroids have been used to treat liver injuries with hypersensitivity features without clear evidence of benefit; therefore they are not recommended routinely to treat drug-induced hepatotoxicity.[9] The only documented benefit of corticosteroids in patients with drug-induced liver disease is methyldopa and nitrofurantoin-associated liver injury, which are both autoimmune hepatitis. Ursodeoxycholic acid may be used to treat cholestatic injuries from drug use, such as terbinafine-induced cholestasis. Pruritus associated with drug-induced cholestatic injury also may be treated with ursodeoxycholic acid.

The management of patients who are taking drugs known to be associated with hepatotoxicity and who have developed mild elevations in liver enzymes can be problematic, as assessing the potential for severe liver injury may be difficult. Many drugs associated with mild elevations in liver enzymes can be continued safely with ongoing and frequent clinical monitoring. The drug should be discontinued promptly if a steady increase in liver enzymes is observed. Avoiding drugs known to be hepatotoxic in patients with multiple risk factors for drug-induced liver disease also can decrease the risk of liver injury. When the cause of hepatic injury is uncertain or the drug is essential for the well-being of the patient, a rechallenge with the drug can be attempted safely.[32] A rechallenge is relatively safe if the hepatotoxicity is cholestatic, but may be dangerous if the injury is hepatocellular necrosis. A safe rechallenge with a potentially hepatotoxic drug involves administration of a single dose and observing the liver enzymes for several days thereafter. The drug can be initiated safely on a routine basis if no change occurs with close monitoring of the liver enzymes for the duration of the drug therapy.

There are several reported cases of cross-hepatotoxicity between drugs within the same class, such as NSAIDs, macrolides, sulfonamides, tricyclic antidepressants, and phenothiazine derivatives.[18] In most cases, the cause of liver injury is the metabolite and not the parent compound. If the drug is essential for the patient, and the use of the drug within the same class is considered, the similarity to the chemical structure of the offending drug should be assessed carefully to better estimate the possibility of cross-reactivity.[32] Drugs associated with enzyme induction or inhibition can produce drug-drug interactions when administered concomitantly with substrates of the interactions and can result in liver injury. Potential for severe drug–drug interactions should be assessed, especially in older individuals who are on multiple drug therapy and more susceptible to drug hepatotoxicity. Follow-up liver enzyme concentrations should be monitored routinely for drugs known to be associated with liver injury.

IMPLICATIONS FOR NURSING PRACTICE

Nurses involved in the direct care and monitoring of patients with potential drug-induced liver disease should be diligent in assessing the signs and symptoms of liver injury and recommending liver function tests for those patients on drugs with predictable hepatotoxicity. Nurses should be aware of drugs likely to cause liver injuries and be educated on recognizing the signs and symptoms of liver injury associated with drug use. The most recent drugs reported to cause liver injuries and which have received warnings issued by the US Food and Drug Administration (FDA) include duloxetine and orlistat. The elderly are especially susceptible to hepatic injury because of age-associated changes in drug metabolism and possible multiple drug regimens. This population can benefit from the nurses who provide care and are able to recognize potential cases of drug-induced liver toxicity. The most important role for all health care professionals, including nurses, in preventing drug-induced liver disease is reporting all potential cases of drug-induced liver injuries to ongoing adverse drug reaction surveillance organizations or to the FDA. The National Institutes of Health have created the Drug-Induced Liver Injury Network to develop a standardized method of identifying and characterizing drug-induced hepatotoxicity. Accurate assessment of adverse events and frequency of occurrence through postmarketing surveillance can help prevent future drug-induced liver injuries.

SUMMARY

Drug-induced liver disease is a common occurrence and an important clinical problem. With more than 1000 drugs implicated in causing liver disease and a growing number of offending drugs, identifying and preventing drug-induced liver injury are challenging tasks for health care providers. Drug-induced liver injury can resemble all forms of acute and chronic liver disease. Although most cases resolve upon withdrawal of the causative agent, there remain numerous cases of fatal hepatotoxicity and of liver injuries requiring liver transplantation. Nurses have a prominent role in recognizing and monitoring drug-induced liver disease in susceptible patients with multiple risk factors. Nurses need to acquire a general knowledge on risk factors for drug-induced liver disease and common clinical features associated with the spectrum of liver diseases associated with drug use. Furthermore, it is important to be able to recognize drugs that are known to cause hepatotoxicity. Prevention is the key to approaching drug-induced liver disease, and effective communication with other health care professionals is crucial in providing patient care with positive clinical outcomes.

REFERENCES

1. Zimmerman HJ. Drug-induced liver disease. Clin Liver Dis 2000;4:73–96.
2. Lee WM. Drug-induced hepatotoxicity. N Engl J Med 2003;349:474–85.
3. Pugh AJ, Barve AJ, Falkner K, et al. Drug-induced hepatotoxicity or drug-induced liver injury. Clin Liver Dis 2009;13(2):277–94.
4. Larrey D. Epidemiology and individual susceptibility to adverse drug reactions affecting the liver. Semin Liver Dis 2002;22:145–55.
5. Sgro C, Clinard F, Ouazir K, et al. Incidence of drug-induced hepatic injuries: a French population-based study. Hepatology 2002;36:451–5.
6. Friis H, Andreasen PB. Drug-induced hepatic injury: an analysis of 1,100 cases reported to the Danish committee on adverse drug reactions between 1978 and 1987. Intern Med 1992;232:133–8.
7. Ostapowicz G, Fontana RJ, Schiodt FV, et al. Results of a prospective study of acute liver failure at 17 tertiary care centers in the United States. Ann Intern Med 2002;137:947–54.
8. Shapiro MA, Lewis JH. Causality assessment of drug-induced hepatotoxicity: promises and pitfalls. Clin Liver Dis 2007;11:477–505.
9. Kaplowitz N, DeLeve LD. Drug-induced liver disease. 2nd edition. New York: Informa Healthcare; 2007.
10. Zimmerman HJ, Ishak KG. Valproate-induced hepatic injury: analyses of 23 fatal cases. Hepatology 1982;2:591–7.
11. Garcia Rodriguez LA, Williams R, Derby LE, et al. Acute liver injury associated with nonsteroidal anti-inflammatory drugs and the role of risk factors. Arch Intern Med 1994;154:311–6.
12. Prescott LF. Paracetamol, alcohol, and the liver. Br J Pharmacol 1999;49:291–301.
13. Gunawan BK, Kaplowitz N. Mechanisms of drug-induced liver disease. Clin Liver Dis 2007;11:459–75.
14. Drug-induced liver injury: review article. Dig Dis Sci 2007;52:2463–71.
15. McJunkin B, Barwick KW, LIttle WC, et al. Fatal massive hepatic necrosis following acetaminophen overdose. JAMA 1976;236(16):1874–5.
16. Ramachandran R, Kakar S. Histological patterns in drug-induced liver disease. J Clin Pathol 2009;62:481–92.
17. Lewis JH. Drug-induced liver disease. Med Clin North Am 2000;84:1275–311.
18. Larry D. Drug-induced liver diseases. J Hepatol 2000;32(Suppl 1):77–88.
19. Valla D, Le MG, Poynard T, et al. Risk of hepatic vein thrombosis in relationship to recent use of oral contraceptives. A case control study. Gastroenterology 1986; 90:807–11.
20. Yu MC, Yuan JM. Environmental factors and risk for hepatocellular carcinoma. Gastroenterology 2004;127(Suppl 5):S72–8.
21. Maheshwari S, Sarraj A, Kramer J, et al. Oral contraception and the risk of hepatocellular carcinoma. J Hepatol 2007;47(4):506–13.
22. Stedman C. Herbal toxicity. Semin Liver Dis 2003;22:195–206.
23. Valla D, Benhamou JP. Drug-induced vascular and sinusoidal lesions of the liver. Clin Gastroenterol 1988;2:481–500.
24. Horowitz RS, Feldhaus K, Dart RC. The clinical spectrum of Jin Bu Huan toxicity. Arch Intern Med 1996;156:899–903.
25. Humberston CL, Akhtar J, Krenzelok EP. Acute hepatitis induced by kava kava. J Toxicol Clin Toxicol 2003;41:109–13.
26. Pak E, Esrason KT, Wu VH. Hepatotoxicity of herbal remedies: an emerging dilemma. Prog Transplant 2004;14:91–6.

27. Sarma DN, Barrett ML, Chavez ML, et al. Safety of green tea extracts: a systematic review by the US Pharmacopeia. Drug Saf 2008;31(6):469–84.
28. Larson AM. Acetaminophen hepatotoxicity. Clin Liver Dis 2007;11:525–48.
29. Perry HE, Shannon WM. Efficacy of oral versus intravenous N-acetylcysteine in acetaminophen overdose: results of an open-label clinical trial. J Pediatr 1998; 132:149–52.
30. Buckley NA, Buckely N, Whyte IM, et al. Oral or intravenous N-acetylcysteine: which is the treatment of choice for acetaminophen (paracetamol) poisoning? J Toxicol Clin Toxicol 1999;37:759–67.
31. Kanter MZ. Comparison of oral and i.v. acetylcysteine in the treatment of acetaminophen poisoning. Am J Health Syst Pharm 2006;63:1821–7.
32. Boyer TD. Management of the patient with drug-induced liver disease. In: Kaplowitz N, DeLeve LD, editors. Drug-induced liver disease. 2nd edition. New York: Informa Healthcare; 2007. p. 346–52.

Drug Dosing Considerations for the Critically Ill Patient with Liver Disease

Sonia Lin, PharmD, BCPS[a,b,*], Brian S. Smith, PharmD, BCPS[c]

KEYWORDS

• Drug dosing • Liver failure • Child-Pugh • Pharmacokinetics

Critically ill patients often suffer disease processes that can lead to a number of physiologic changes.[1] These changes can lead to alterations in various pharmacokinetic drug parameters affecting the efficacy or safety of medications.[2] Hepatic dysfunction is present in 11% to 54% of critically ill patients depending on the definition used and what critically ill population is being studied.[3–5] Impairment of liver function can alter many different aspects of a drug's pharmacokinetics, including drug absorption, distribution, metabolism, and excretion. This article reviews the pharmacokinetic changes that can occur in hepatic failure, identifies practical ways to quantify the severity of dysfunction, and discusses general drug dosing strategies in this patient population.

PHARMACOKINETIC CHANGES IN LIVER DISEASE
Absorption

Absorption is the process of a drug crossing a biologic membrane before it enters the systemic circulation. Enteric absorption is the most common route of medication administration, but other routes of administration involving absorption include inhalation and subcutaneous, topical, intramuscular, and intraperitoneal administration. Bioavailability describes the fraction of a drug reaching the systemic circulation. Drugs

[a] Department of Pharmacy Practice, College of Pharmacy, University of Rhode Island, 41 Lower College Road, Fogarty Hall, Room 27, Kingston, RI 02881, USA
[b] Department of Pharmacy, UMass Memorial Medical Center, 55 Lake Avenue North, Worcester, MA 01655, USA
[c] Education and Clinical Services, UMass Memorial Medical Center, 55 Lake Avenue North, Worcester, MA 01655, USA
* Corresponding author. Department of Pharmacy Practice, College of Pharmacy, University of Rhode Island, 41 Lower College Road, Fogarty Hall, Room 27, Kingston, RI 02881.
E-mail address: SLin@uri.edu

Crit Care Nurs Clin N Am 22 (2010) 335–340
doi:10.1016/j.ccell.2010.04.006
0899-5885/10/$ – see front matter © 2010 Elsevier Inc. All rights reserved.

administered by the intravenous (IV) route are considered to have a bioavailability of 1, or 100%, indicating that 100% of the dose is reaching the systemic circulation. For this reason, many critically ill patients will receive medications by the IV route initially to ensure the full dose is reaching the systemic circulation. Although IV administration may be preferred in critically ill patients, some medications may be available only in oral dosage forms. In addition, oral administration is generally less costly and may be desirable in patients as their clinical status improves and preparations are made to consolidate or eliminate IV access for transfer out of the intensive care unit.

One of the most significant mechanisms by which hepatic dysfunction can affect the bioavailability of enterally administered drugs is by reducing the first-pass effect. The first-pass effect describes the initial hepatic metabolism of enterally administered medications. In healthy individuals, enterally administered drugs are absorbed through the small intestines into the hepatic portal circulation. The drugs then must pass through the liver before reaching the systemic circulation. This "first-pass" through the liver provides an opportunity for the liver to metabolize and inactivate/eliminate the drug before it reaches the systemic circulation. The extraction ratio for a specific drug will determine the extent of the "first-pass" effect. Additional discussion of extraction ratio will occur later in the article when metabolism is reviewed. Patients with hepatic dysfunction may have reduced ability to metabolize drugs by the first-pass effect. A reduction in the first-pass effect results in a larger amount of the enterally administered drug reaching the systemic circulation, hence increased bioavailability. Common critical care drugs that exhibit an increased bioavailability in hepatic dysfunction with enteral administration include labetolol, metoprolol, midazolam, morphine, nifedipine, and propranolol.[6–11] Caution should be used when starting these medications in patients with hepatic dysfunction. Clinicians should consider starting these medications at a lower dose and carefully monitor for side effects.

Hepatic dysfunction and critical illness have the potential to alter the absorption of enterally administered medications by other mechanisms. Alterations to gastrointestinal motility may alter the rate and extent of absorption. Delayed gastric emptying may result in a delayed time to absorption of medications from the small intestine. Diarrhea may decrease intestinal transit time, limiting the absorption of medications. Hemodynamic instability or the use of vasopressors may reduce the blood flow to the gastrointestinal tract and reduce the absorption of enterally administered medications. Although many factors associated with critical illness may alter the absorption of medications, most pharmacokinetic studies are conducted in healthy subjects or in subjects with stable hepatic dysfunction. As a result, there is an overall lack of data on the influence of hepatic dysfunction and critical illness on medication absorption.

Volume of Distribution

Volume of distribution (Vd) describes a theoretical or calculated volume that a drug is dissolved in. It is calculated by dividing the dose of a drug by the resulting peak serum concentration. For example, if 10 mg of drug X results in a serum concentration of 1 mg/L, the Vd would be 10 L (10 mg divided by 1 mg/L equals 10 L). Drugs that reside primarily in the serum tend to have low volume of distribution and are generally more hydrophilic. Drugs that move out of the serum and into body tissues (brain, adipose, muscle) will generally have a large Vd and are often lipophilic. Hepatic dysfunction or critical illness can cause significant changes in fluid balance in the body. Patients will often retain fluid as part of their disease process. This added fluid could increase the Vd of some medications, especially hydrophilic medications that tend to have a low Vd. As a result, these medications may result in lower plasma concentrations and thus decreased therapeutic efficacy.

Many medications are bound to plasma proteins. Albumin is the most common plasma protein that medications are bound to. Medications with high binding to albumin exist in the serum in a bound form (the drug bound to albumin) or a free form (drug that is not bound to albumin). The free drug is available to exert its pharmacologic action. If a patient has a low albumin level (common in patients with liver disease owing to reduced hepatic production), this can result in a larger amount of free drug, predisposing the patient to exaggerated pharmacologic effects and/or side effects. Common drugs used in critically ill patients who have high protein binding include phenytoin, mycophenolate mofetil, and benzodiazepines such as diazepam, lorazepam, and midazolam.[12–16] When using these drugs in a critically ill patient with hepatic dysfunction, an assessment of the patient's albumin level should be made and lower doses should be considered with monitoring of drug levels where appropriate.

Metabolism/Elimination

Hepatic dysfunction can potentially have an impact on all aspects of drug pharmacokinetics. Because the liver is the main site for drug biotransformation, it is intuitive that this may be altered when hepatic function is impaired. The degree of alteration depends on the degree of hepatic dysfunction and how the liver processes the drug. A drug's extraction ratio, intrinsic hepatic clearance (CL_i), and blood flow to the liver are the primary factors controlling hepatic drug metabolism. The extraction ratio represents the efficiency of the liver to clear a specific drug from the bloodstream as it passes through the liver. The metabolism of drugs with a high extraction ratio is dependent on hepatic blood flow since metabolism is dependent on delivery of drug to the liver. As discussed with the "first-pass" effect, drug bioavailability can also be influenced by the extraction ratio. CL_i represents the liver's intrinsic ability to metabolize a specific drug and is independent of hepatic blood flow.[17]

Drugs can be grouped into categories based on their extraction ratio. High extraction drugs are more than 60% removed on first pass through the liver, resulting in an overall bioavailability of 40% or less.[18] In cirrhosis, there is often an impairment of hepatic blood flow; this can decrease the extent of metabolism of high extraction drugs leading to significantly higher drug exposure. The presence of porto-systemic shunts, which relieve portal pressures as a therapeutic strategy for variceal bleeding in patients with cirrhosis,[19] diverts blood flow away from the liver, also resulting in decreased drug metabolism.[20,21] In contrast, low extraction drugs are not significantly removed ($\leq$30%) on first pass through the liver, resulting in an overall bioavailability of 70% or more. Drug clearance is dependent on the degree of protein binding and its CL_i, rather than hepatic blood flow. Thus, cirrhosis has limited effect on bioavailability of these drugs. However, cirrhosis does have an effect on metabolic CL_i of low extraction drugs. In those with low protein binding, CL_i decreases as hepatic failure advances to cirrhosis because of decreased activity of metabolic enzymes. In those with high protein binding ($\geq$90%), CL_i actually increases as hepatic failure progresses. Hypoalbuminemia is associated with liver disease, which leads to increased free fraction and metabolism of unbound drug.[17]

Changes in other pharmacokinetic parameters can also occur, although not directly as a consequence of liver failure, but indirectly from the common complications that are associated with liver failure. Hepatorenal syndrome and cholestasis can also occur as a result of liver failure. Consequently, renal and biliary drug excretion can be markedly impaired. Finally, activity of specific drug-metabolizing enzymes can be affected by the presence of cholestasis, thus having an additive effect on decreased CL_i.[22]

HEPATIC FUNCTION ASSESSMENT

Drug pharmacokinetics have the potential to be significantly changed in critically ill patients with hepatic dysfunction. As discussed in this article, alterations in absorption, distribution, metabolism, and elimination can occur. Clinicians providing care to critically ill patients need to appreciate the potential change that hepatic dysfunction can have on a drug's pharmacokinetic profile to anticipate and prevent medication misadventures. Unfortunately, there is currently no single marker or test routinely available to clinicians to accurately determine what extent hepatic dysfunction will have on a drug's pharmacokinetics. Dynamic liver function tests using specific compounds or probes, which can be measured with serial drug levels, can precisely quantify the metabolic capacity of specific enzymes in the liver. However, these tests are not routinely available to clinicians and many are not practical for use in routine care. As a result, clinicians will generally use less sensitive tools to provide guidance. The most common way to assess hepatic function for use in drug dosing is the Child-Pugh classification.[23] The Child-Pugh classification assigns points based on a patient's serum bilirubin, serum albumin, prothrombin time, presence of encephalopathy, and presence of ascites. Based on the number of points, the patient is classified as having mild (5–6 points), moderate (7–9 points), or severe (10–15 points) disease. Although this tool was not developed for drug-dosing adjustments, many drug-dosing recommendations in the package insert for drugs recommend dose reduction or avoiding use of the medication based on the Child-Pugh score.

When providing care to critically ill patients with hepatic dysfunction, a clinician must have a solid understanding of a drug's pharmacokinetic properties, in combination with an assessment to changes in the patient's physiology. The following are a few general recommendations related to drug dosing in hepatic dysfunction.

1. When possible, avoid medications that undergo significant hepatic metabolism. If the medication is eliminated by the kidneys, an adequate assessment of renal function should be made.
2. If a medication has available dosing recommendations or guidelines, such as based on a Child-Pugh classification score, these dosing recommendations should be considered.
3. When dosing recommendations or guidelines do not exist, calculation of a Child-Pugh score can still be helpful. Assessment of the patient's bilirubin, albumin, and prothrombin time can provide useful information about the functional status of the liver.
4. Starting with lower doses of medications and slowly titrating the dose up based on response is recommended. Specific monitoring plans are also recommended to determine if the patient is reaching his or her therapeutic goals or experiencing side effects.
5. When appropriate or applicable, serum drug monitoring should be performed.
6. Careful risk/benefit analysis must be conducted when starting medications with serious side effects and/or narrow therapeutic index.
7. When in doubt, individuals with advanced training in drug pharmacokinetics and drug metabolism should be consulted in designing drug regimens (hepatologists, clinical pharmacists).

SUMMARY

Hepatic dysfunction in the critically ill patient presents a unique challenge to clinicians when designing pharmacotherapeutic treatment plans. Overall, the literature regarding drug dosing in critically ill patients with hepatic dysfunction is incomplete and current tools available to bedside clinicians have limitations. Despite these challenges, rational drug regimens can be implemented by critical care nurses who consider the potential impact of hepatic dysfunction on drug pharmacokinetics. This information can be applied clinically and careful monitoring plans can be implemented to assess a drug for efficacy and safety.

REFERENCES

1. McKindley DS, Hanes S, Boucher BA. Hepatic drug metabolism in critical illness. Pharmacotherapy 1998;18(4):759–78.
2. Boucher BA, Wood GC, Swanson JM. Pharmacokinetic changes in critical illness. Crit Care Clin 2006;22(2):255–71.
3. Kramer L, Jordan B, Druml W, et al. Incidence and prognosis of early hepatic dysfunction in critically ill patients—a prospective multicenter study. Crit Care Med 2007;35(40):1099–104.
4. Kortgen A, Paxian M, Werth M, et al. Prospective assessment of hepatic function and mechanisms of dysfunction in the critically ill. Shock 2009;32(4):358–65.
5. Power BM, Millar Forbes A, van Heerden PV, et al. Pharmacokinetics of drugs used in critically ill adults. Clin Pharm 1998;34(1):25–56.
6. Homeida M, Jackson L, Roberts CJ. Decreased first-pass metabolism of labetalol in chronic liver disease. Br Med J 1978;2:1048–50.
7. Regardh CG, Jordo L, Jundborg P, et al. Pharmacokinetics of metoprolol in patients with hepatic cirrhosis. Clin Pharm 1981;6:375–88.
8. Pentikainen PJ, Valisalmi L, Himberg JL, et al. Pharmacokinetics of midazolam following intravenous and oral administration in patients with chronic liver disease and in healthy subjects. J Clin Pharmacol 1989;29:272–7.
9. Hasselstrom J, Eriksson S, Persson A, et al. The metabolism and bioavailability of morphine in patients with severe liver cirrhosis. Br J Clin Pharmacol 1990;29: 289–97.
10. Kleinbloesem CH, van Harten J, Wilson JP, et al. Nifedipine: kinetics and hemodynamic effects in patients with liver cirrhosis after intravenous and oral administration. Clin Pharmacol Ther 1986;40:21–8.
11. Branch RA, Kornhauser DM, Shand DG, et al. Biological determinants of propranolol disposition in normal subjects and patients with cirrhosis. Br J Clin Pharmacol 1977;4:630.
12. Perucca E. Free level monitoring of antiepileptic drugs clinical usefulness and case studies. Clin Pharm 1984;9:71–8.
13. Nowak I, Shaw LM. Mycophenolic acid binding to human serum albumin: characterization and relation to pharmacodynamics. Clin Chem 1995;41:1011–7.
14. Kober A, Jenner A, Sjoholm I, et al. Differentiated effects of liver cirrhosis on albumin binding sites for diazepam, salicylic acid and warfarin. Biochem Pharmacol 1978;27:2729–35.
15. Wilkinson GR. The effects of liver disease and aging on the disposition of diazepam, chlordiazepoxide, oxazepam, and lorazepam in man. Acta Psychiatr Scand 2007;58:56–74.
16. Trouvin JH, Farainotti R, Haberer JP, et al. Pharmacokinetics of midazolam in anaesthetized cirrhotic patients. Br J Anaesth 1988;60:762–7.
17. Bauer LA. Clinical pharmacokinetics and pharmacodynamics. In: DiPiro JT, Talbert RL, Yee GC, et al, editors. Pharmacotherapy: a pathophysiologic approach. 7th edition. New York: McGraw-Hill; 2008. p. 9–30.

18. Delco F, Tchambaz L, Schlienger R, et al. Dose adjustment in patients with liver disease. Drug Saf 2005;28(6):529–48.
19. Sease JM, Timm EG, Stragand JJ. Portal hypertension and cirrhosis. In: DiPiro JT, Talbert RL, Yee GC, et al, editors. Pharmacotherapy: a pathophysiologic approach. 7th edition. New York: McGraw-Hill; 2008. p. 633–49.
20. Pomier-Layrargues G, Huet PM, Villeneuve JP, et al. Effect of portacaval shunt on drug disposition in patients with cirrhosis. Gastroenterology 1986;91(1):163–7.
21. Ohkubo H, Okuda K, Lida S, et al. Role of portal and splenic vein shunts and impaired hepatic extraction in the elevated serum bile acids in liver cirrhosis. Gastroenterology 1984;86(3):514–20.
22. Tanaka M, Nakura H, Tateishi T, et al. Ursodeoxycholic acid prevents hepatic cytochrome P450 isozyme reduction in rats with deoxycholic acid-induced liver injury. J Hepatol 1999;31:263–70.
23. Pugh RN, Murray-Lyon IM, Dawson JL, et al. Transection of the oesophagus for bleeding oesophageal varicies. Br J Surg 1973;60:646–9.

Current and Emerging Strategies for Treating Hepatic Encephalopathy

Keith J. Foster, PharmD, BCPS[a], Sonia Lin, PharmD, BCPS[b,*], Charles J. Turck, PharmD, BCPS[c]

KEYWORDS

- Hepatic encephalopathy • Lactulose • Probiotics
- Acarbose • L-carnitine • Flumazenil

Hepatic encephalopathy (HE) is a constellation of metabolic derangements stemming from hepatic impairment and culminating in neuropsychiatric dysfunction.[1–5] Experts have formulated 2 classification systems that describe the range of etiologies and disease severity engendered by HE. One system is from the World Congress of Gastroenterology, which stratifies the causes of HE into 3 major categories: "*A*" for acute liver failure; "*B*" for portal-systemic shunts, in the absence of intrinsic hepatic insufficiency, that bypass the liver and its detoxifying role; and "*C*" for cirrhosis together with either portal-systemic shunts or portal hypertension.[6] The other system, the West Haven Criteria, is an ordinal scoring system describing the continuum of HE severity, ranging from Grade 1, in which the patient exhibits mild cognitive impairment, to Grade 4, in which the patient becomes comatose. The severity of liver disease may be predictive of HE development,[3] and risk factors include dehydration, constipation, renal failure, sodium and potassium imbalances, infections, gastrointestinal hemorrhage, and hepatocellular carcinoma.[3,4]

Although there is a wide spectrum of HE severity, even milder forms of HE adversely impact patients' quality of life.[7–9] Liver disease and HE may precipitate sleep disorders,[10] impair learning and memory,[11] and deprive patients of their autonomy by affecting motor functions from as simple as walking to as complex as driving.[8,9]

[a] Surgical Intensive Care Unit, Department of Pharmacy, UMass Memorial Medical Center, 55 Lake Avenue North, Worcester, MA 01655, USA
[b] UMass Memorial Medical Center, 55 Lake Avenue North, Worcester, MA 01655, USA
[c] Surgical Intensive Care Unit, Department of Pharmacy, UMass Memorial Medical Center, 119 Belmont Street, Worcester, MA 01605, USA
* Corresponding author. Department of Pharmacy Practice, University of Rhode Island, College of Pharmacy, 27 Fogarty Hall, Kingston, RI.
E-mail address: SLin@uri.edu

Crit Care Nurs Clin N Am 22 (2010) 341–350
doi:10.1016/j.ccell.2010.04.007
0899-5885/10/$ – see front matter © 2010 Elsevier Inc. All rights reserved.

Almost 15% of patients die while awaiting a liver transplant, and 58% of patients with severe HE die within 1 year.[12]

PATHOGENESIS

Although various chemicals are implicated in HE, it is classically described[1-4] as arising from the liver's inability to convert ammonia (NH_3) to urea. NH_3 accumulates in the brain, disrupting neurochemical function and eventually manifesting as a change in mental status. Situations that allow NH_3-rich blood to avoid the liver's metabolic effect may contribute to HE, including damage to the liver in diseases like cirrhosis[6]; the development of portacaval shunts, which is common in patients with chronic liver disease[13,14]; or the surgical placement of portosystemic shunts in patients with cirrhosis[15] and transplant[16] patients.

Astrocytes, the star-shaped glial cells that help maintain the structural integrity of the central nervous system (CNS) and blood-brain barrier (BBB), are key players in reducing NH_3 levels in the CNS by drawing on the chemical to synthesize glutamate to glutamine.[1,17] On onset of hyperammonianemia, glutamine accumulates in the astrocytes,[18] ultimately leading to an alteration of the structural integrity of the BBB and the potentially overt neuropsychological function.[1,11]

In recent decades, there has been an increasing appreciation for the role that the other neurotoxins play in HE, including hepatic excretion of the trace element manganese, which plays a mediating role with the excitatory neurotransmitter glutamate[4]; and the inability to metabolize phenols[19] and sulfuric by-products[2,5,9,20] from amino acid breakdown in the gastrointestinal (GI) tract. The patient with hepatic insufficiency is also unable to metabolize several chemical by-products of vegetable digestion that mimic the inhibitory effects of the benzodiazepine (BZ) drug class.[4]

CLINICAL MANIFESTATIONS

The classic clinical manifestations of HE comprise a wide variety of neuropsychiatric, neurophysiological, and neurologic symptoms depending on the severity of the disease.[21] The most common changes seen are in the level of consciousness, and in intellectual and neuromuscular function. Changes in consciousness may include subtle changes in personality, sleep-wake cycle and, in later stages of severity, lethargy, stupor, or coma.[21] Changes in intellectual function may include unusual behavior, disorientation to time and place, decreased memory, and confusion.[21] The most common neuromuscular disturbance is a flapping tremor called asterixis.[21] Asterixis is the loss of agonist and antagonist regulation of muscle tone, resulting in an inability to maintain posture. The flapping tremor can be demonstrated by instructing a patient to maintain their arms outstretched with wrists dorsiflexed and fingers spread open. An abrupt loss in flexor tone and a wrist drop in a periodic manner every 2 to 3 seconds is a characteristic sign. One can also look for other signs such as loss of tone in the tongue, pedal dorsiflexion, and fist clenching. Asterixis is usually not present in a comatose patient, so testing for abnormal eye movements, the development of a pyramidal syndrome, and decerebrate posturing[22] would be more helpful in the diagnosis of HE. A pyramidal tract dysfunction includes hypertonia, hyperreflexia, and extension plantar responses, which may later be replaced by hypotonia when coma develops.[21] Additional neuromuscular signs may include the development of a mild parkinsonism characterized by bradykinesia with or without tremor, ataxia, and dsyarthria.[23] The presence of seizures is questionably related to HE, and may be more common in patients who are withdrawing from alcohol or are suffering from a drug-induced or metabolic syndrome.[24]

Additional laboratory and physical findings may be present, with severe hepatic dysfunction.[22] The findings include muscle wasting, jaundice, ascites, palmar erythema, and spider telangiectasias. Muscle wasting, spider telangiectasias, and palmar erythema usually develop over time, and are typically not present in the acute phase. Visual disturbances, most likely resulting from the cortical and reticular dysfunction associated with an increase in NH_3 levels, have been documented.[25] Reticular dysfunction has been termed "hepatic retinopathy" and is associated with damage to the retinal glia or Muller cells. Fetor hepaticus, a sweet musty breath that smells like rum, can be observed in patients with liver failure and those with portosystemic shunts regardless of the presence of HE.[26]

Minimal hepatic encephalopathy (MHE) is a newer classification of HE that is characterized by subtle changes in daily living, including decreased energy level, disruption of normal sleep-wake cycle, and impairment of cognition, consciousness, motor function, attention, and cooperation.[6] Subtle motor changes include increased tone, reduced speed or clumsiness of rapid alternating movements, ataxia, increased deep tendon reflexes, or impairment of positive or postural reflexes. As a result, patients may have significant impairment in performing complex functional activities such as driving. MHE is a major cause of early retirement and has a detrimental effect on health-related quality of life.[27]

DIAGNOSIS

A clinical evaluation is generally sufficient to diagnose HE.[22] In most cases, imaging studies, neurophysiologic testing, and biochemical markers are not necessary. Imaging studies such as computed tomography scan, magnetic resonance imaging, and magnetic resonance spectroscopy can be used to differentiate HE from diagnoses such as hemorrhage, abscess or tumor, and intracerebral infarctions.[22] Neurophysiological testing, such as the electroencephalographic (EEG) P300-evoked potential and the critical flicker frequency test, may help in detection of MHE. Neuropsychologic testing, such as number connection test parts A (NCT-A) and B (NCT-B), the digit symbol test, and the block design test are used to evaluate attention, concentration, and memory. Alterations in biochemical markers in hepatic failure include hypoalbuminemia, prolonged prothrombin time, elevated liver function tests, and thrombocytopenia. Although these markers are not specific to HE, they can be used to help confirm the clinical diagnosis.

MANAGEMENT OF PRECIPITATING FACTORS

Initial management of HE should include identification and treatment of precipitating factors. Well-recognized factors include high protein diet, gastrointestinal bleeding, electrolyte imbalances, infection, and constipation.[21] The role of nutrition in preventing HE is discussed in article by Zhao and Ziegler elsewhere in this issue. Gastrointestinal hemorrhage is a major cause for patients to develop symptoms. Treatment generally consists of screening the patient for *Helicobacter pylori* infection, administering proton pump inhibitors, and providing endoscopic intervention if necessary. The use of antibiotics is warranted in patients with known variceal bleeds or for those requiring treatment for a spontaneous bacterial perotinitis.[5] Early treatment has been shown to improve outcomes. Electrolyte imbalances such as hyponatremia and hypokalemia have been shown to increase the risk of developing HE by altering the effects of NH_3 on astrocytes.[5] The use of neuroactive agents, such as opioid analgesics, may exacerbate episodes of HE by mechanisms beyond that of just suppressing neurologic function. These agents are known to cause constipation, especially after long-term use, which is a risk factor for developing HE symptoms. The use of laxatives and enemas, in conjunction with a diet that is high in fiber, may be beneficial in relieving constipation.[28]

PHARMACOLOGIC THERAPY

Most pharmacologic treatment options for HE aim at decreasing NH_3 levels, either by reducing NH_3 production or facilitating NH_3 excretion. Some of the emerging therapies target alternate pathogenetic pathways.

Nonabsorbable Disaccharides

Lactulose is a nonabsorbable disaccharide used in the treatment of HE because of its effects on reducing blood NH_3 levels. Lactulose is fermented by bacteria in the colon, resulting in the production of fatty acids and various gases and a decrease in colon pH. Acidification of the colon (to pH 5–5.5) results in NH_3 being drawn out of the portal circulation and converted into ammonium (NH_4^+) ion, which is poorly reabsorbed from the GI tract. The trapped ammonium ions are excreted with feces, and this leads to decreased blood NH_3 levels.[29,30] Lactitol, another nonabsorbable disaccharide, has a similar effect to lactulose on colonic pH.[31] It is considered more palatable than lactulose, but is only available in Europe.

Lactulose can be administered orally for chronic encephalopathy in doses of 15 to 45 mL (containing 10–30 g lactulose) 3 to 4 times daily; the dose is adjusted to achieve 2 to 3 semi-soft bowel movements per day. An increased frequency of administration of hourly doses is used initially in acute encephalopathy, and doses may be administered via nasogastric tube or rectally in patients who cannot tolerate oral administration.[28] Adverse effects are mainly gastrointestinal related: diarrhea, abdominal pain, nausea, and flatulence. Lactulose is available commercially as a solution (10 g per 15 mL),[32] as well as crystal packets for oral reconstitution (10 g per packet).[33]

Although lactulose is considered as first-line drug therapy in the management of HE,[28] a systematic review of the existing literature conducted by Als-Nielsen and colleagues[34] does not support this practice. An overall positive effect of lactulose on HE (compared with placebo or no treatment) was observed if the results of all studies were taken collectively. However, this effect was not sustained when only high-quality studies were considered. In addition, lactulose did not seem to have any beneficial effect on mortality.

Lactulose may still play an important role in the treatment of HE. In a study conducted by Prasad and colleagues,[35] patients with cirrhosis having MHE who were treated for 3 months with lactulose showed significant improvement in neuropsychologic testing when compared with those who did not receive treatment. More importantly, lactulose-treated patients demonstrated significant improvements across various dimensions of the Sick Impact Profile, a questionnaire used to evaluate health-related quality of life.

Antibiotics

Because of the pathogenic origin of NH_3, antibiotics can be used as an alternative therapy to nonabsorbing disaccharides for the management of HE. Certain antibiotics decrease the concentration of NH_3-producing bacteria in the colon, which in turn leads to lower blood NH_3 levels. Antibiotics may also decrease blood concentrations of BZ-like compounds that are also produced by gut bacteria.[28,36] The various antibiotics that have been evaluated for this indication and reported to have similar efficacy to lactulose include neomycin, paromomycin, metronidazole, and rifaximin. The adverse effects associated with long-term use limits the use of these antibiotics. As discussed later, rifaximin may have slight advantages over other drug therapies.[36]

Neomycin is a poorly absorbed aminoglycoside antibiotic that has previously been widely used for HE. In addition to reducing bacterial load in the colon, it can also inhibit glutaminase activity in the intestinal mucosa. Doses of 1 to 2 g per day are recommended for chronic HE. Dose recommendations for acute HE are higher, at 3 to 6 g/d for a 1- to 2-week period.[28] The most commonly used regimen in clinical trials was 1 g 3 times daily for 14 to 21 days.[37] Although only a small amount of the drug is systemically absorbed, use of neomycin is limited by auditory loss and renal failure with prolonged therapy. Annual auditory screening and periodic monitoring of kidney parameters should be conducted with chronic therapy.[38] Neomycin is commercially available as an oral solution (125 mg/5 mL) and 500-mg tablets.[39]

Metronidazole is an antibiotic with activity against gram-negative anaerobes with similar efficacy to neomycin in the treatment of HE.[28,40] Doses should be initiated at 250 mg twice daily and adjustments should be made for hepatic impairment.[41] Routine use of metronidazole is limited by its potential neurotoxicity, particularly in patients with cirrhosis.[42] Concomitant administration with alcohol can lead to symptoms characterized by flushing, vomiting, headache, and abdominal discomfort.[36]

Rifaximin is a rifamycin-derived antibacterial agent with broad-spectrum activity against aerobic and anaerobic, gram-positive and gram-negative organisms.[43] It is poorly absorbed with the majority of the drug being eliminated in the feces, allowing it to remain in the GI tract at its intended site of action. Significant drug interactions have not been reported with rifaximin, and its dose need not be adjusted for renal or hepatic dysfunction, making it an attractive treatment alternative for HE.

Dosage for optimal lowering of NH_3 levels in blood and reducing severity of encephalopathy was found to be 1200 mg per day, administered as 400 mg 3 times daily. Treatment duration ranges from 14 to 21 days. Rifaximin is commercially available as a 200-mg tablet and does not have a generic equivalent.[44]

In clinical trials, rifaximin has been shown to be as effective as, if not more effective than, nonabsorbable disaccharides and other antibiotics in lowering blood NH_3 levels and improvement in severity of asterixis, intellectual function, EEG abnormalities, overall severity of encephalopathy, and mental status.[37,45] When compared with lactulose, rifaximin had a more significant and sustained impact on the desired outcomes in a shorter period of time.[46,47] Rifaximin was also better tolerated than lactulose. Final conclusions of comparative efficacy with lactulose should be taken with a grain of salt, because the doses of lactulose used in these comparative studies were not maximized, which leads to bias toward the efficacy of rifaximin. Rifaximin seems to be equally as effective as paromomycin. When compared with neomycin, rifamixin may have an advantage in lowering of NH_3 levels,[48] earlier normalization of EEG,[49] and overall tolerability.[48]

Although rifamixin is effective in treating HE and seems to be more effective as well as better tolerated than some existing therapies, there are reservations in adopting it as a first-line treatment alternative. Antimicrobial resistance is not a problem at present, but could potentially arise in the future.[50] Rifaximin is more expensive than lactulose. Based on a recent decision analysis evaluating the cost-effectiveness of various initial treatment regimens for HE,[51] lactulose monotherapy provided the optimal cost per quality-adjusted life-year gained (QALY-gained). Alternatively, if rifaximin was used as a treatment option for patients who failed to improve on optimized lactulose doses, a minimal increase in cost per QALY-gained was seen. Therefore, rifaximin should be reserved for use only in patients who fail lactulose monotherapy.

Probiotics

Because NH_3 is produced by gut microflora, the administration of probiotics to modify natural intestinal flora may be considered as an additional treatment alternative for HE.[52] Probiotic products such as Synbiotic 2000 (contains 4 probiotic species and 4 prebiotics) and products containing *Enterococcus faecium* SF68 alone, *Bifidobacterium longum* alone, and a combination of *Streptococcus faecalis*, *Clostridium butyricum*, *Bacillus mesentericum*, and lactic acid bacillus have all been shown to have beneficial effects.[52–54] Probiotics showed improvement in neuropsychological function tests after daily doses for 30 to 60 days. Daily intake of 12 ounces of yogurt containing live *Lactobacillus* species, *S thermophilus*, and *Bifidobacteria* for 60 days has also been shown to be of some benefit with improvements in NCT-A, block design, and digit symbol tests.[55] When compared with lactulose, use of probiotics containing *E faecium* SF68 alone and *B longum* alone resulted in significantly greater improvement in outcomes.[53,56]

L-Carnitine

L-Carnitine is an endogenous NH_3 compound thought to have therapeutic value in HE because of different mechanisms. These mechanisms include being a cofactor in the oxidation of fatty acids in mitochondria, participating in the production of ketone bodies, and facilitating the transfer of acetyl coenzyme A (CoA) from mitochondria to cytoplasm.[57] The transfer of acetyl CoA is essential in the production of acetylcholine. Three studies, all from the same center and investigators, showed the potential benefit of L-carnitine in HE. The first 2 studies consisted of patients with subacute to moderate HE symptoms and showed the superiority of 4 g of oral carnitine over placebo. The total number of patients in the first 2 studies was 120, and serum NH_3 concentrations and the NCTs were used as end points for these studies.[58] The results showed an improvement in serum NH_3 levels of 40.75 μM/L versus 5.75 μM/L for carnitine versus placebo, respectively. For the NCT score, an improved mean of 21.9 seconds faster than placebo was shown in the carnitine population. The third study comprised 150 patients in all stages of West Haven criteria and showed similar results in the lower stages of disease (Stages 0, 1, and 2). However, in a small subset of patients with hepatic coma, there seemed to be a worsening of Glasgow Coma scoring (5.9, 95% confidence interval 2.72–6.68).[57]

Acarbose

Acarbose is an antidiabetic agent that inhibits α-glucosidases at the intestinal brush border, inhibiting glucose absorption. In addition, it may also have effects on promoting intestinal saccharolytic flora. A study conducted by Gentile and colleagues[59] demonstrated that treatment with acarbose, 100 mg 3 times daily for 8 weeks, in patients with cirrhosis with grade 1 to 2 HE and concomitant type 2 diabetes resulted in significantly lower NH_3 levels and improved intellectual function scores than patients who received placebo. Fasting and postprandial glucose levels were also significantly decreased, which is to be expected. Based on the results of this study, the use of acarbose therapy as an alternative therapy for HE should be limited to patients with concomitant diabetes mellitus.

Flumazenil

Flumazenil is a drug that acts as an antagonist toward the BZ–γ-aminobutyric acid (GABA) receptor complex located in the brain. It has been proposed that patients with cirrhosis and HE have increased endogenous BZ or BZ-like substances, which can bind to this receptor complex and lead to neuroinhibitory effects from activation of the GABA portion of the receptor complex.[28,60]

The efficacy of flumazenil was evaluated by Barbaro and colleagues[61] in a large, multicenter, double-blind, placebo-controlled cross-over study. Patients (n = 527) with grade III and IVa HE were included in this study. Patients who were assigned to the treatment group received flumazenil 1 mg intravenously, in addition to lactulose 30 mL every 6 hours. Significant improvements were seen in neurologic scores (based on a modified Glasgow Coma Scale) and EEG tracings after 3 hours in patients treated with flumazenil. Of the patients with grade III HE at baseline, 17.5% demonstrated improved neurologic scores as compared with 3.8% in the placebo group. The corresponding numbers among the patients with grade IVa HE were 14.7% versus 2.7%, respectively. With respect to EEG tracings, 27.8% of patients with grade III HE and 21.5% of patients with grade IV HE showed improvements with flumazenil compared with 5% and 2% with placebo, respectively. When outcomes of this study were combined collectively with other studies evaluating the use of flumazenil versus placebo, similar results were seen.[60] A significantly greater proportion of patients in the treatment group showed an improvement in EEGs, as well as overall clinical improvement (decrease in EEG and clinical neurologic function; grading method different across studies included).

The specific role of flumazenil in the treatment of HE has not been defined. Existing practice guidelines recommend its use be reserved for patients with acute HE, in conjunction with BZ use.[28] Flumazenil is only commercially available as an injectable solution of 0.1 mg/mL,[62] thus its use in chronic, mild encephalopathy is limited.

SUMMARY

Various treatment options exist for the management of HE, but lactulose remains the gold standard. Alternative and emerging therapies such as rifaximin, probiotics, L-carnitine, acarbose, and flumazenil may be used in patients who do not respond to or cannot tolerate lactulose. Critical care nurses need to have a working knowledge of the efficacy and toxicity of these different agents because they play a major role in assessing the patients' response to therapy.

REFERENCES

1. Jalan R, Shawcross D, Davies N. The molecular pathogenesis of hepatic encephalopathy. Int J Biochem Cell Biol 2003;35:1175–81.
2. Butterworth RF. Pathophysiology of hepatic encephalopathy: a new look at ammonia. Metab Brain Dis 2002;4:221–7.
3. Munoz SJ. Hepatic encephalopathy. Med Clin North Am 2008;92:795–812.
4. Sundaram V, Shaikh OS. Hepatic encephalopathy: pathophysiology and emerging therapies. Med Clin North Am 2009;93:819–36.
5. Wright G, Jalan R. Management of hepatic encephalopathy in patients with cirrhosis. Best Pract Res Clin Gastroenterol 2007;21:95–100.
6. Ferenci P, Lockwood A, Mullen K, et al. Hepatic encephalopathy—definition, nomenclature, diagnosis, and quantification: final report of the Working Party at the 11th World congresses of Gastroenterology, Vienna. Hepatology 1998;35: 716–21.
7. Amodio P. Health related quality of life and minimal hepatic encephalopathy. It is time to insert 'quality' in health care. J Gastroenterol Hepatol 2009;24:329–30.
8. Blendis L. Hepatic encephalopathy forward to the past. Gastroenterology 2006; 130:2239–40.

9. Bajaj JS. Minimal hepatic encephalopathy matters in daily life. World J Gastroenterol 2008;14:3609–15.
10. Mostacci B, Ferlisi M, Baldi Antognini A, et al. Sleep disturbance and daytime sleepiness in patients with cirrhosis: a case control study. Neurol Sci 2008;29: 237–40.
11. Ahboucha S, Butterworth RF. The neurosteroid system: implication in the pathophysiology of hepatic encephalopathy. Neurochem Int 2008;52:575–87.
12. Childers JW, Arnold RM. Hepatic encephalopathy in end-stage liver disease #188. J Palliat Med 2008;11:1341–2.
13. Olde Damink SWM, Jalan R, Dejong CHC. Interorgan ammonia trafficking in liver disease. Metab Brain Dis 2009;24:169–81.
14. Riggio O, Efrati C, Catalona C, et al. High prevalence of spontaneous portal-systemic shunts in persistent hepatic encephalopathy: a case-control study. Hepatology 2005;42:1158–64.
15. Deng D, Liao MS, Qin JP, et al. Relationship between pre-TIPS hepatic hemodynamics and postoperative incidence of hepatic encephalopathy. Hepatobiliary Pancreat Dis Int 2006;5:232–6.
16. Braun MM, Bar-Nathan N, Shaharabani E, et al. Postshunt hepatic encephalopathy in liver transplant recipients. Transplantation 2009;87:734–9.
17. Albrecht J, Norenberg MD. Glutamine: a Trojan horse in ammonia neurotoxicity. Hepatology 2006;44:788–94.
18. Lavoie J, Giguère JF, Pomier Layrargues G, et al. Amino acid changes in autopsied brain tissue from cirrhotic patients with hepatic encephalopathy. J Neurochem 1987;49:692–7.
19. Gerber T, Schomerus H. Hepatic encephalopathy in liver cirrhosis. Pathogenesis, diagnosis and management. Drugs 2000;60:1353–70.
20. Wendon J, Lee W. Encephalopathy and cerebral edema in the setting of acute liver failure: pathogenesis and management: Neurocrit Care 2008;9:97–102.
21. Jones EA, Weissenborn K. Neurology and the liver. J Neurol Neurosurg Psychiatry 1997;63:279–93.
22. Weissenborn K. Diagnosis of encephalopathy. Digestion 1998;59(Suppl 2):22–4.
23. Lizardi-Cervera J, Almeda P, Guevara L, et al. Hepatic encephalopathy: a review. Ann Hepatol 2003;2(3):122–30.
24. Ficker DM, Westmoreland BF, Sharbrough FW. Epileptiform abnormalities in hepatic encephalopathy. J Clin Neurophysiol 1997;14:230–4.
25. Eckstein AK, Reichenbach A, Jacobi P, et al. Hepatic retinopathia. Changes in retinal function. Vision Res 1997;37:1699–706.
26. Mitchell S, Ayesh R, Barrett T, et al. Trimethylamine and foetor hepaticus. Scand J Gastroenterol 1999;34:524–8.
27. Ortiz M, Jacas C, Cordoba J. Minimal hepatic encephalopathy: diagnosis, clinical significance and recommendations. J Hepatol 2005;42(Suppl 1):S45–53.
28. Blei AT, Cordoba J. Hepatic encephalopathy: practice guidelines. Am J Gastroenterol 2001;96:1968–76.
29. Avery GS, Davies EF, Brogden RN. Lactulose: a review of its therapeutic and pharmacologic properties with particular reference to ammonia metabolism and its mode of action of portal systemic encephalopathy. Drugs 1972;4(1):7–48.
30. Clausen MR, Mortensen PB. Lactulose, disaccharides and colonic flora. Clinical consequences. Drugs 1997;53(6):930–42.
31. Patil DH, Westaby D, Mahida YR, et al. Comparative modes of action of lactitol and lactulose in the treatment of hepatic encephalopathy. Gut 1987;28: 255–9.

32. Lactulose [package insert]. Lexi-drugs, Lexi-comp, Inc, 2009.
33. Kristalose® Prescribing Information. Nashville (TN): Cumberland Pharmaceuticals; 2006.
34. Als-Nielsen B, Gluud LL, Gluud C. Non-absorbable disaccharides for hepatic encephalopathy: systematic review of randomized trials. BMJ 2004;328:1046–50.
35. Prasad S, Dhiman RK, Duseja A, et al. Lactulose improves cognitive functions and health-related quality of life in patients with cirrhosis who have minimal hepatic encephalopathy. Hepatology 2007;45(3):549–59.
36. Festi D, Vestito A, Mazzella, et al. Management of hepatic encephalopathy: focus on antibiotic therapy. Digestion 2006;73(Suppl 1):94–101.
37. Lawrence KR, Klee JA. Rifaximin for the treatment of hepatic encephalopathy. Pharmacotherapy 2008;28(8):1019–32.
38. Neomycin. In: DRUGDEX® System [Internet database]. Greenwood Village, CO: Thomson Reuters (Healthcare) Inc. Updated periodically.
39. Neomycin [package insert]. Lexi-drugs, Lexi-Comp, Inc, 2009.
40. Morgan MH, Read AE, Speller DCE. Treatment of hepatic encephalopathy with metronidazole. Gut 1982;23:1–7.
41. Loft S, Sonne J, Døssing M, et al. Metronidazole pharmacokinetics in patients with hepatic encephalopathy. Scand J Gastroenterol 1987;22(1):117–23.
42. Uhl MD, Riely CA. Metronidazole in treating portosystemic encephalopathy. Ann Intern Med 1996;124(4):455.
43. Adachi J, DuPont HL. Rifaximin: a novel nonabsorbed rifamycin for gastrointestinal disorders. Clin Infect Dis 2006;42:541–7.
44. Xifaxan prescribing information. Salix Pharmaceuticals, Inc, 2008.
45. Maclayton DO, Eaton-Maxwell A. Rifaximin for treatment of hepatic encephalopathy. Ann Pharmacother 2009;43:77–84.
46. Bucci L, Palmieri CG. Double-blind, double-dummy comparison between treatment with rifaximin and lactulose in patients with medium to severe degree hepatic encephalopathy. Curr Med Res Opin 1993;13:109–18.
47. Massa R, Vallerino E, Dodero M. Treatment of hepatic encephalopathy with rifaximin: double-blind, double-dummy study versus lactulose. Eur J Clin Res 1993;4:4–18.
48. Pedretti G, Calzetti C, Missale G, et al. Rifaximin versus neomycin on hyperammonemia in chronic portal systemic encephalopathy of cirrhosis: a double-blind, randomized trial. Ital J Gastroenterol 1991;23:175–8.
49. Festi D, Mazzella G, Orsini M, et al. Rifaximin in the treatment of chronic hepatic encephalopathy: results of a multicenter study of efficacy and safety. Curr Ther Res Clin Exp 1993;54:598–609.
50. Alcorn J. Review: rifaximin is equally or more effective than other antibiotics and lactulose for hepatic encephalopathy. ACP J Club 2008;149(5):11.
51. Huang E, Esrailian E, Spiegel BMR. The cost-effectiveness and budget impact of competing therapies in hepatic encephalopathy—a decision analysis. Aliment Pharmacol Ther 2007;26:1147–61.
52. Sheth AA, Garcia-Tsao G. Probiotics and liver disease. J Clin Gastroenterol 2008; 42(Suppl 2):S80–4.
53. Malaguarnera M, Gargante MP, Malaguarnera G, et al. Bifidobacterium combined with fructo-oligosaccharide versus lactulose in the treatment of patients with hepatic encephalopathy. Eur J Gasteroenterol Hepatol 2010;22(2): 199–206.
54. Sharma P, Sharma BC, Puri V, et al. An open-label randomized controlled trial of lactulose and probiotics in the treatment of minimal hepatic encephalopathy. Eur J Gastroenterol Hepatol 2008;20:506–11.

55. Bajaj JS, Saeian K, Christensen KM, et al. Probiotic yogurt for the treatment of minimal hepatic encephalopathy. Am J Gastroenterol 2008;103:1707–15.
56. Loguercio C, Abbiati R, Rinaldi M, et al. Long-term effects of *Enterococcus faecium* SF68 alone versus lactulose in the treatment of patients with cirrhosis and grade 1 to 2 hepatic encephalopathy. J Hepatol 1995;23:39–46.
57. Shores NJ, Keeffe EB. Is oral l-acetyl-carnitine an effective therapy for hepatic encephalopathy? Review of the literature. Dig Dis Sci 2008;53:2330–3.
58. Malaguarnera M, Pistone G, Astuto M, et al. L-carnitine in the treatment of mild or moderate hepatic encephalopathy. Dig Dis 2003;21:271–5.
59. Gentile S, Guarine G, Romano M, et al. A randomized controlled trial of acarbose in hepatic encephalopathy. Clin Gastroenterol Hepatol 2005;3(2):184–91.
60. Goulenok C, Bernard B, Cadranel JF, et al. Flumazenil vs. placebo in hepatic encephalopathy in patients with cirrhosis: a meta-analysis. Aliment Pharmacol Ther 2003;16:361–72.
61. Barbaro G, Di Lorenzo G, Soldini M, et al. Flumazenil for hepatic encephalopathy Grade III and IVa in patients with cirrhosis: an Italian multicenter double-blind, placebo-controlled, cross-over study. Hepatology 1998;28:374–8.
62. Flumazenil [package insert]. Bedford Laboratories, 2007.

Hepatorenal Syndrome: A Comprehensive Overview for the Critical Care Nurse

James N. Fleming, PharmD, BCPS[a],*, Ahmad Abou Abbass, MD[b]

KEYWORDS

- Hepatorenal • Syndrome • Renal failure • Cirrhosis
- Nurse • Critical care

An association between advanced liver disease, ascites, and oliguric renal failure was originally noted in the 1860s. Later, in an article published in 1956, Hecker and Sherlock[1] described 9 patients in whom progressive renal dysfunction was accompanied by worsening systemic circulation. These patients were treated with intravenous noradrenalin (NA, ie, norepinephrine), temporarily improving systemic blood pressure and increasing urine output, although all eventually succumbed. Interestingly, on postmortem biopsy of the patients' kidneys, the investigators noted that there were no significant histologic changes to the kidneys. Based on their observations, the investigators hypothesized that the cause of the progressive renal failure was peripheral arterial vasodilation.[1] This was later described as "hepatorenal syndrome" (HRS) and the pathophysiology and definition have been elucidated over the following half-century. It has further been discovered that in addition to having no histologic changes associated with the renal failure, the kidneys' tubular function was preserved and the condition was reversible. This was best demonstrated by cases in which kidneys from donors with hepatorenal syndrome were successfully transplanted into patients with end-stage renal failure, and was supported by an early report of 3 patients who recovered from HRS after successful liver transplantation.[2,3]

None of the authors have any financial relationships to disclose.
[a] Solid Organ Transplant, Department of Pharmacy Services, Henry Ford Hospital, 2799 West Grand Boulevard, Detroit, MI 48202, USA
[b] Division of Transplant, Henry Ford Hospital, 2799 West Grand Boulevard, Detroit, MI 48202, USA
* Corresponding author.
E-mail address: jflemin2@hfhs.org

DEFINITION AND DIAGNOSIS

The definition of HRS was originally determined by expert consensus in Rome, Italy, in 1978. The historic diagnosis primarily focused on a rising serum creatinine (SrCr) greater than 1.5 mg/dL in the presence of liver disease and absence of hypovolemia or response to a fluid load. It was further updated and outlined by the International Ascites Club (IAC) in 1996 and then again in 2007.[4,5] The most current definition of HRS is a potentially reversible syndrome that occurs in patients with cirrhosis, ascites, and liver failure, as well as patients with acute liver failure or alcoholic hepatitis. It is characterized by impaired renal function, marked alterations in cardiovascular function, and overactivity of the sympathetic nervous and renin-angiotensin system.[5] The 2007 IAC Diagnostic Criteria are seen in **Box 1**. The main differences from the 1996 criteria are as follows: (1) creatinine clearance has been excluded because it is more complicated than serum creatinine and does not increase the accuracy of renal function estimation; (2) renal failure in the setting of ongoing bacterial infection, but in absence of septic shock, is now considered HRS; (3) plasma volume expansion should be performed with albumin rather than saline based on IAC member opinion that it causes more and longer expansion than saline; and (4) the minor diagnostic criteria have been removed because they are not essential.[5]

As can be seen, the diagnosis of HRS is still a diagnosis of exclusion. Risk factors for renal impairment, such as shock, overdiuresis, and use of nephrotoxic medications must be ruled out. It must be proven the renal failure is not caused by intravascular depletion. This requires a cessation of diuretics and plasma expansion with albumin.

HRS is classified into 2 different clinical types: type 1 and type 2 HRS.

Type 1 Hepatorenal Syndrome

Type 1 HRS is a rapidly progressive renal failure defined by a doubling of the initial SrCr to a level of greater than 2.5 mg/dL occurring within 2 weeks of baseline. This clinical type of HRS is usually caused by a precipitating factor and carries a poor prognosis.[4–6]

Box 1
2007 International Ascites Club's diagnostic criteria of hepatorenal syndrome

Cirrhosis with accumulation of ascites

Low glomerular filtration rate, as indicated by serum creatinine of >1.5 mg/dL

No improvement of serum creatinine (decrease to a level of 1.5 mg/dL or less) after at least 2 days with diuretic withdrawal and volume expansion with albumin. The recommended dose of albumin is 1 g/kg of body weight per day up to a maximum of 100 g/d

No current or recent treatment with nephrotoxic drugs (ie, aminoglycosides, nonsteroidal anti-inflammatory drugs)

Absence of shock

Absence of parenchymal kidney disease

This can be identified by proteinuria >500 mg/d, microhematuria (>50 red blood cells per high-powered field), and/or abnormal renal ultrasonography

Data from Salerno F, Gerbes A, Gines P, et al. Diagnosis, prevention, and treatment of hepatorenal syndrome in cirrhosis. Postgrad Med J 2008;84:662–70.

Type 2 Hepatorenal Syndrome

Type 2 HRS is a progressive, steady renal failure with a SrCr greater than 1.5 mg/dL. Whereas type 1 HRS classically has a precipitating factor, type 2 HRS may have a precipitating factor but frequently occurs spontaneously. It characteristically occurs in patients with refractory ascites.[5,6]

PATHOPHYSIOLOGY

The mechanism by which the diseased liver affects renal function has never been fully understood. Early investigations in the 1960s and 1970s showed that HRS was associated with significant renal vasoconstriction. Although the renal vasoconstriction historically was thought to differ from low-output cardiac failure because of the high cardiac output (CO) in patients with cirrhosis, it has been determined in light of both old evidence from Tristani and Cohn[7] and more recently by Ruiz-del-Arbol and colleagues[8,9] that patients with lower CO are more likely to develop HRS. This helps demonstrate that, although CO can be low, normal, or high, it is insufficient for the patient's needs because of reduced peripheral resistance.[5] "Cirrhotic cardiomyopathy," characterized by blunted systolic and diastolic responses to stimuli, or a decreased venous return in patients are a few hypotheses of the mechanism leading to insufficient CO in patients developing HRS.[5] The most recent investigations have focused on determining the factors involved in the intense renal vasoconstriction. Some of these factors include the renin-angiotensin-aldosterone system (RAAS),[10] sympathetic nervous system (SNS),[11] and renal prostaglandins.[12] Four interrelated pathways have been implicated in the pathophysiology of HRS.[6] Each patient's renal vasoconstriction is mediated by variable degrees of each of these 4 pathways:

1. Peripheral arterial vasodilation with hyperdynamic circulation and subsequent renal vasoconstriction
2. Stimulation of the renal sympathetic nervous system
3. Cardiac dysfunction contributing to the circulatory derangements and renal hypoperfusion
4. Action of cytokines and vasoactive mediators on the renal circulation and other vascular beds.

Peripheral Arterial Vasodilation

The "peripheral arterial vasodilation hypothesis" of sodium and water retention in cirrhosis, by Schrier and colleagues,[13] well explains the impact of peripheral vasodilation in cirrhosis on the renal vasculature that occurs during HRS. As a result of the increased resistance of blood flow through the cirrhotic liver and vasodilation of the systemic and splanchnic circulation because of increased vasodilator production, there is splanchnic blood pooling leading to a decrease in effective circulating blood volume (ECBV). Because of the decreased ECBV, the high-pressure baroreceptors in the aortic arch and carotid body produce compensatory activation of the SNS, RAAS, and nonosmotic release of vasopressin (antidiuretic hormone [ADH]). This leads to a picture of hyperdynamic circulation with high CO and low systemic vascular resistance (SVR), hypotension, and vasoconstriction of the renal vasculature. As cirrhosis progresses, the splanchnic vasodilation worsens, leading to more compensatory mechanisms and more pronounced vasoconstriction of extrasplanchnic vascular beds, including the kidney.[14]

Stimulation of the Renal SNS

Patients with cirrhosis are known to have increased sympathetic nervous tone.[11] Animal evidence also suggests that a hepatorenal reflex that is activated by an increase in the hepatic sinusoidal pressure or reduction in sinusoidal blood flow exists. In humans, lumbar sympathectomy in 5 patients with HRS and a glomerular filtration rate (GFR) less than 25 mL/min led to an increased GFR, whereas 3 others with GFR greater than 25 mL/min did not demonstrate increased GFR.[15] This suggests that renal sympathetic nerve activity contributes to renal vasoconstriction in a select group of patients with HRS, but does not serve a primary role in all humans with HRS.

Cardiac Dysfunction Contributing to the Circulatory Derangements and Renal Hypoperfusion

As a consequence of the increased CO and heart rate that are the hallmark features of the hyperdynamic circulation present in advanced liver cirrhosis, the impaired myocardial performance in cirrhotic patients can be underestimated. Nevertheless, the constant mechanical stress and exposure to neurohormonal factors cause a condition termed "cirrhotic cardiomyopathy," which includes increased ventricular wall size and systolic and diastolic dysfunction. The mechanism of this impaired cardiac function is complex and incompletely understood, but may include neurohormonal hyperactivity causing myocardium growth, diminished myocardial β-adrenergic receptor signal transduction, and an inhibitory effect of nitric oxide on ventricular function. Torregrosa and colleagues[16] were the first to demonstrate that the worsening of cardiac function in decompensated patients with cirrhosis under stress improves 6 to 12 months after liver transplantation, showing that it is the diseased liver that causes the cardiac dysfunction. Ruiz-del-Arbol and colleagues[8] recently established that impaired cardiac function plays a major role in HRS that results in patients during an episode of spontaneous bacterial peritonitis (SBP). In their study, patients who developed HRS had a significantly reduced CO without a change in SVR at the time of SBP diagnosis compared with those who did not develop HRS. They demonstrated an intense systemic inflammatory response at the time of infection and an inability of these patients to compensate with increased SVR. Cardiac output decreased, however cardiopulmonary pressures and heart rate did not change, suggesting that these patients had decreased venous return. This idea is supported by the fact that infusion of albumin in these patients, and so increasing intravascular volume, significantly reduces the rate of HRS in patients with SBP.[17] These findings possibly identify patients with a decrease in CO as a population at risk for HRS. It may be that these patients have a relatively depressed cardiac response to stress that contributes to their systemic hypotension and renal hypoperfusion.

Cytokines and Vasoactive Mediators

Many factors may be involved in the regulation of intrarenal hemodynamics that differentiate patients with cirrhosis from patients with cirrhosis who develop HRS. Some of the agents studied include nitric oxide (NO), tumor necrosis factor (TNF)-α, endothelin, endotoxin, glucagon, and intrarenal vasodilating prostaglandins.[6] Patients with cirrhosis with ascites have been shown to have higher NO plasma concentrations than patients with compensated cirrhosis. This elevated NO level is associated with a high plasma RAAS activity and ADH in addition to low urinary sodium excretion.[6] It would be expected that elevated NO levels would cause vasodilation of renal arterioles as well. Conversely, vasoconstriction predominates in patients with HRS. Why this occurs is not clear, but it has been proposed that an increase in plasma symmetric dimethylarginine, an endothelial NO synthase inhibitor, in terminal liver failure and accumulation in the renal vasculature may prevent the increased NO level in the renal vasculature and promote renal vasoconstriction in HRS.[18] Patients who develop HRS also have demonstrated a decline in urinary prostaglandin excretion. Because renal vasoconstriction is counterbalanced by vasodilating prostaglandins, this may also be a contributor in HRS. This theory is supported by the evidence that the administration of inhibitors of the enzyme cyclooxygenase (COX), which is responsible for prostaglandin synthesis, to patients with decompensated cirrhosis precipitates a renal failure syndrome that is similar to HRS.[12]

CLINICAL FEATURES

Patients with compensated cirrhosis have increased plasma volume, reduced SVR, and high CO all in the presence of relatively normal arterial pressure. As patients begin to decompensate, they develop renal insufficiency and sodium and water retention and their systemic circulation abnormalities worsen, leading to reduced arterial pressure. Patients with HRS have these same abnormalities, but tend to have more significant arterial hypotension, regardless of an increasing stimulation of the SNS, RAAS, and nonosmotic release of ADH, indicating a progressive impairment in arterial circulation during the progression from compensated to decompensated cirrhosis and to HRS.[4]

Type 1 and type 2 HRS are distinctly different in clinical features. In the first pattern, patients experience rapidly progressive reduction of GFR, with accompanying increases in serum blood urea nitrogen (BUN) and SrCr levels, oliguria, extreme hyponatremia, and hyperkalemia. In these patients with type 1 HRS, the cascade of events is typically triggered by complicating events, such as bacterial infections, gastrointestinal hemorrhage, and surgical procedures. The other subgroup of patients, those with type 2 HRS, typically experience a steady reduction of GFR and accompanying increase in BUN and SrCr that occurs and persists over weeks or months as cirrhosis progresses. Patients experiencing type 2 HRS have much better survival compared with the previous pattern, although these patients can commonly progress into a rapid progressive renal failure in the setting of a complicating event or illness. The same pathogenic mechanisms appear to underlie both clinical scenarios, whereas they differ in the time to progression and intensity.[4]

INCIDENCE

The incidence of HRS has been inconsistent in many large studies. In one early analysis, Gines and colleagues[19] estimated a 1-year incidence of 18% and a 5-year incidence of 39%. This analysis was done before the current IAC's Diagnostic Criteria, however, and so may not provide an accurate estimation. In another analysis of 68 patients with decompensated cirrhosis with multiple risk factors for SBP and HRS, the 1-year incidence of type 1 HRS with 1996 IAC definitions was 30% and type 2 HRS was 3%.[20] This was a high-risk population for HRS, however, and may have higher rates than many other populations.

In 263 patients with decompensated cirrhosis with ascites, Planas and colleagues[21] found a 5-year HRS probability of 11.4% overall (8.9% type 2, 5.4% type 1). This was using the 1996 IAC definition, and is substantially lower than some other reports. The subgroup of patients in this study did not have as advanced liver disease as in some other studies, which may be why their estimation was lower. In this follow-up, the complication with the worst prognosis in this analysis was confirmed to be HRS, similar to others. Patients who developed type 1 HRS had a median survival of

1 week. Patients with type 2 HRS had a somewhat better prognosis, but still had only a 38.5% survival rate at 1 year.

It is clear from the results of these analyses that the incidence of HRS is difficult to determine for patients with cirrhosis in general and is largely dependent on the stage of liver disease and the risk factors present.

RISK FACTORS

Bacterial infections are one of the most common risk factors for type 1 HRS. Of infections, SBP carries with it a 20% to 30% risk. However, timely treatment with adequate antibiotics, such as third-generation cephalosporins, can rapidly reverse HRS in up to 30% of cases.[22] In addition, plasma volume expansion with albumin was shown in one large study to significantly reduce the incidence of renal failure (33% vs 10%) and mortality (41% vs 22%) compared with patients treated with placebo.[17] Furthermore, large-volume paracentesis without albumin replacement for volume expansion has been shown to precipitate HRS in 15% of patients.[23] In 161 patients with upper gastrointestinal bleeds, 11% developed renal failure. These patients tended to have higher Childs-Turcotte-Pugh (CTP) scores and require more blood products than those who did not develop renal failure.[24] Over-diuresis leading to intravascular volume depletion is considered a common risk factor for HRS. As for nephrotoxic medications, nonsteroidal anti-inflammatory drugs (NSAIDs) have been reported to cause renal failure in patients with cirrhosis and ascites by inhibiting renal prostaglandin synthesis, which are important mediators of both afferent and efferent renal arteriolar vasodilation.[11] In one historical review, renal failure occurred in 53% of patients with cirrhosis who were on aminoglycosides[25] (Box 2).

TREATMENT

Although type 2 HRS can usually be managed on an outpatient basis, type 1 HRS is a rapidly progressive syndrome with high mortality that requires hospitalization. Typically, these patients will require intensive monitoring, especially of fluid status. A central venous catheter is ideal to accurately assess intravascular volume via central venous pressure (CVP) monitoring, although this is not always necessary. Immediately all potential causes of renal failure should be withdrawn and triggering factors should be ruled out. This includes stopping diuretics and potentially nephrotoxic medications and performing therapeutic and diagnostic paracentesis on tense ascites. Currently, it is recommended by most experts to provide 25% albumin replacement (8 g/L) for patients with 5 L or more removed by paracentesis.[26] Albumin has been shown to

---

Box 2
Risk factors for type 1 hepatorenal syndrome

Bacterial infections (especially SBP)

Large-volume paracentesis without concentrated (25%) albumin replacement

Gastrointestinal bleeds

Overdiuresis

NSAIDs

Aminoglycosides

be more effective than crystalloids at preventing renal failure after large-volume para-centesis and is superior to other plasma expanders.[23,27] Although not backed by controlled trials, it is also suggested to put the patient on free water restriction and a low-salt diet to aid in reducing ascites and preventing reaccumulation after para-centesis.[26] Once these general supportive measures are implemented, the patient should be assessed for overall prognosis. If it is deemed that the patient is a potential candidate for liver transplantation, aggressive therapy for type 1 HRS is indicated. If not deemed suitable for transplantation, the patient has a very poor prognosis and further therapy is unlikely to be effective. The 4 major therapeutic interventions for HRS are (1) pharmacologic treatment, (2) renal replacement therapy (RRT), (3) TIPS, and (4) liver transplantation (**Box 3**).

Box 3
Management of type 1 hepatorenal syndrome

General Management

Intensive fluid status monitoring

  CVP monitoring if possible

Withdraw potential causes of renal failure

  Diuretics

  Nephrotoxic medications

Free water restriction and low-salt diet

Therapeutic and diagnostic paracentesis of tense ascites

  Concentrated albumin replacement if ≥5 L removed

  Timely initiation of antibiotic therapy (third-generation cephalosporins) and 25% albumin for SBP

Assess prognosis and suitability for liver transplantation

Pharmacologic Management

Vasoconstrictors

  Terlipressin 0.5–1.0 mg IV every 4–6 hours (may be increased to maximum 12 mg/d)

  Midodrine 7.5 mg + Octreotide 100 μg every 8 hours (may be increased to 15 mg and 200 μg)

  Noradrenalin (norepinephrine) 0.5–3.0 mg per hour

  Vasopressin (doses not standardized)

Albumin 1 mg/kg (up to 100 g), then 25–40 g/d may increase response to vasoconstrictors (hold if CVP >18 mm Hg or serum albumin >4.5 mg/dL)

Renal Replacement Therapy

  Intermittent hemodialysis

  Continuous renal replacement therapy

  Molecular adsorbent recirculating system

Surgical Management

Transjugular intrahepatic portosystemic shunt

Definitive Therapy

Liver transplantation

Pharmacologic Treatment

The goal of pharmacologic treatment is to reverse or prevent renal failure and prolong survival until the patient can receive a liver transplant. Renal vasodilators and systemic vasoconstrictors are the 2 main types.

Renal vasodilators

The use of renal vasodilators was based on the hypothesis that it would antagonize the intensive renal vasoconstriction that is the acute cause of HRS. Although it was historically hypothesized that "renal-dose dopamine" (RDD) (2–3 μg/kg/min) infusions should selectively cause vasodilation of the renal arterioles and increase renal blood flow (RBF), this therapy has been shown to have no impact on the GFR or urine flow either alone or in combination with prostaglandins.[28,29] Although RDD did show some effect in combination with norepinephrine and ornipressin, respectively, these results can be attributed to the concomitantly administered therapy.[30,31] Thus, use of renal vasodilators in the treatment of HRS has been abandoned.

Systemic vasoconstrictors

Systemic vasoconstrictors are theorized to work based on reversing the splanchnic vasodilation present in patients with HRS. This improves circulatory function and ECBV and so improves renal perfusion and GFR by reversal of the intense renal vasoconstriction. The vasoconstrictors that have been most studied and will be included in this article are vasopressin analogs, somatostatin analogs, and α-adrenergic agonists.

Vasopressin analogs are agonistic of the V1 receptors on arterial wall smooth muscles, producing significant vasoconstriction. Ornipressin has been shown to have beneficial effects on renal function in combination with RDD, albumin, and alone[31–33]; however, the high rates of ischemic complications have limited its use in clinical practice.

Terlipressin was designed with the aim of producing a vasopressin (VP) analog with lower toxicity. It is a hormonogen of lysine-VP (3 glycyl residues and a lysine-VP) that has 1 amino acid difference from arginine-VP (ADH). Lysine-VP has a higher affinity for smooth muscle V1 receptors over renal V2 receptors than arginine-VP (ratio of 2.2 vs 1.0). Following intravenous bolus administration, the glycyl residues are cleaved by endothelial peptidases allowing a slow, prolonged release of lysine-VP over 4 to 6 hours.[34] In clinical studies for HRS, it has been given as intravenous (IV) boluses ranging 0.5 to 2.0 mg/dose every 4 to 12 hours for up to 15 days. In the largest randomized study to date, 1 mg IV every 6 hours was used with an increase up to 2 mg IV every 6 hours if the SrCr did not decrease by 30% or more by day 3 of therapy.[35] Terlipressin has shown improved urine output (UO), GFR, mean arterial pressure (MAP), and reduced SrCr in more than 50% of patients with coadministration of albumin in both retrospective analyses and prospective trials.[36–39] Patients with type 2 HRS appear to have a higher response rate compared with patients with type 1 HRS in the studies that allowed their inclusion (see **Box 4** for definitions of response rates). It appears that patients who have less severe liver disease (CTP score <13) are more likely to have a clinical response.[36] It also appears from one small report that terlipressin is more efficacious when administered with albumin than without.[39] Because of this, most recent studies use terlipressin in addition to concentrated albumin 1 mg/kg on day 1 of therapy and then 25 to 40 g per day every day afterward titrated to CVP between 15 and 18 cm H_2O.[35,40] An expert consensus statement allows that, in patients in which CVP monitoring is not necessary, albumin may be given and discontinued only if serum albumin is greater than 4.5 mg/dL or in the case of pulmonary edema.[5] Although albumin appears to improve the clinical

---

Box 4
Definitions of response to therapy

Complete response – Reduction in SrCr ≤1.5 mg/dL

Partial response – Reduction in SrCr by ≥50% of pretreatment value without reaching 1.5 mg/dL

Relapse – recurrence of renal failure after discontinuation of therapy (SrCr >1.5 mg/dL)

Nonresponse – No decrease to <50% of pretreatment value

Data from Salerno F, Gerbes A, Gines P, et al. Diagnosis, prevention, and treatment of hepatorenal syndrome in cirrhosis. Postgrad Med J 2008;84:662–70.

---

response to terlipressin, albumin alone is not as efficacious, proving that replacing ECBV is not enough.[40] About 17% to 50% of patients will recur into HRS, but usually respond to resuming administration (Colle I).[36,39] This calls into question the duration of terlipressin administration. Because all studies to this point have limited treatment to 15 consecutive days, it is unknown what effect a longer duration of therapy would have. Experts recommend a maximum therapy of 14 days. They also advise that if a reduction in SrCr does not occur within 3 days or if there is not a 50% decrease within 7 days, terlipressin therapy may be abandoned.[5] Adverse effects in these clinical studies have been mild compared with ornipressin, with ischemic complications occurring in less than 10% of patients and in most studies no different than placebo. One of the largest current drawbacks for terlipressin is its unavailability in much of the world, including the United States. Although it has been used in Europe for more than 20 years, it has only recently been used to any degree in the United States. The Food and Drug Administration (FDA) granted terlipressin Orphan Drug status in 2004, and then upgraded it to Fast Track status in 2005. As of 2008, it has been approved for a rolling New Drug Application (NDA) submission. One of the main studies that supported this status was an international, multicenter, randomized, prospective, double-blind, placebo-controlled trial in 112 patients performed in the United States, Germany, and Russia.[35] In this study, the investigators demonstrated that terlipressin was significantly more effective than placebo at reversing HRS according to the commonly held definition of improvement of SrCr to 1.5 mg/dL or less (see **Box 4**). The results were especially robust in patients who received at least 3 days of therapy with terlipressin. Despite the efficacy of reversing HRS, patient mortality is still up to 80% at 3 weeks and without liver transplantation, 80% of responders will die within 3 months.[36] This is because terlipressin does nothing to change the underlying liver disease. Successful treatment of HRS before liver transplantation, however, has demonstrated an improvement in survival after liver transplantation.[41]

Another vasoconstrictor that has been studied in patients with HRS is the oral α_1 agonist, midodrine. Midodrine is a prodrug that is rapidly deglycinated after absorption into its active metabolite, desglymidodrine, a potent α_1 agonist, causing an increase in vascular tone in both the arterial and venous vasculature. Midodrine on its own has shown little effect in patients with HRS. This may be because of an impaired response to arterial vasoconstrictors. This response is related to an increase in both endothelial (prostacyclin and NO) and nonendothelial vasodilators (glucagon). Studies have shown that inhibition of glucagon can normalize the arterial response.[42,43] With this information, it was hypothesized that midodrine may be efficacious in combination with octreotide, a synthetic analog of somatostatin, and a natural inhibitor of glucagon release. Most studies have used a starting dose of midodrine 5.0 or 7.5 mg orally every 8 hours along with octreotide 100 μg subcutaneously every 8 hours and the ability to increase the dosages to 12.5 or 15.0 mg and 200.0 μg 3 times daily of midodrine and octreotide, respectively, with a goal increase in MAP of 15 mm Hg in addition to standard therapy. Although small (15–60 patients), all of these studies have shown a significant increase in MAP, GFR, UO, and 1-month survival (60% to 80% vs 16% to 30%) compared with low-dose dopamine or current standard supportive care. The therapy has also been continued for up to 2 months and was able to be taken as an outpatient.[42,44] Adverse events were minimal.

Arginine vasopressin infusion has been widely used in patients with HRS but without many large clinical trials supporting its use. In one retrospective study including 43 patients receiving vasopressin infusions, octreotide infusions, or both, vasopressin infusion or vasopressin plus octreotide was associated with a significantly higher response compared with octreotide infusion alone (42% vs 38% vs 0%) and had a significantly better survival and liver transplant rate.[45] The average dosage of vasopressin used in the patients who responded, however, was about 0.23 units per minute. This dose is 5 times higher than "physiologic dose vasopressin," which is used in some patients with sepsis (0.04 units per minute). Although no adverse events were confirmed in this retrospective study, dosages this high of vasopressin in other populations has led to significant rates of cardiac and mesenteric ischemia.[46]

Noradrenalin (NA) is a catecholamine with predominately α-adrenergic receptor agonism, causing significant peripheral vasoconstriction without significant vasoconstriction of the coronary arteries. In an early pilot study, Duvoux and colleagues[47] treated 12 patients with a NA infusion beginning at 0.5 mg/h (~8 μg/min) and titrated to improve the MAP by 10 mm Hg and increase 4-hour UO to greater than 200 mL. The infusion could last up to 15 days and could be reintroduced for patients who relapse through treatment. The infusion reversed HRS in 83% of the patients after 7 days, on average. It is notable that 2 of the patients who responded to NA had previously failed terlipressin therapy. Two of the 12 patients experienced chest pain with NA, and 1 of the patients had an echocardiogram demonstrating hypokinesia at the left ventricular apex, which disappeared with NA withdrawal. With these early encouraging results, a larger randomized pilot study was performed in Italy. In this study 22 patients were randomized to either terlipressin 1 mg IV every 4 hours with increase to 2 mg IV every 4 hours if no response by 3 days (12 patients) or NA infusion starting at 0.10 μg/kg/min and then titrated up by 0.05 μg/kg/min every 4 hours with a maximum of 0.70 μg/kg/min to achieve an increase in MAP by 10 mm Hg (10 patients) for a maximum of 2 weeks. This study showed similar efficacy in regard to reversal of HRS between NA and terlipressin (70% and 83%, respectively). Recurrence of HRS, liver transplantation rates, and survival were not significantly different between the groups and there were no recorded ischemic events.[48] In a later study with 40 patients using NA 0.5 to 3.0 mg/h compared with terlipressin, response rates and survival were identical between groups and consistent with the previous reports.[49] These encouraging results probably signify that patients' endogenous catecholamines are unable to increase their SVR to the degree necessary to improve ECBV, probably because of the impaired arterial reactivity to vasopressors in patients with cirrhosis. With pharmacologic-dose NA, the ECBV is improved, homeostatic vasoactive systems are suppressed, and renal blood flow is improved. This is supported by the reduction in the RAAS activity seen with administration of NA and terlipressin and the reduction in norepinephrine concentrations seen in patients treated with terlipressin.[37,47,49] Because of the similar efficacy, wider availability, and lower cost as compared with terlipressin, further study may help identify NA as an adequate alternative for treatment of hospitalized patients with type 1 HRS.

Systemic vasoconstrictors are a very promising therapy for management of HRS as a bridge to transplantation. Future study will hopefully identify the most effective agents and regimens.

Transjugular Intrahepatic Portosystemic Shunt

The transjugular intrahepatic portosystemic shunt (TIPS) is an angiographically created shunt between the portal and hepatic venous systems placed through the hepatic parenchyma. The patency of the shunt is maintained using an expandable metal stent. TIPS works by effectively decompressing the portal system and reducing portal pressures. It does so by acting as a side-to-side portocaval shunt without the need for major surgery.[50] TIPS has been studied extensively in the management of complications from cirrhosis and portal hypertension, such as the management of variceal bleeding and refractory ascites.[51–54] TIPS has been shown to result in improvement in renal function in patients with refractory ascites. It reduces the portal pressure and returns pooled blood to systemic circulation, increasing the ECBV, down-regulating the RAAS, and inhibiting renal vasoconstriction.[55–57] A few case reports and preliminary data suggest that TIPS may improve renal function in the setting of HRS.[58–62] These studies have mainly included patients with relatively preserved hepatic function and a CTP of 11 or lower. This excludes many patients with HRS who have advanced liver disease. TIPS also comes with complications. One of the main problems is shunt thrombosis or stenosis, which requires frequent reinterventions, although the more recent use of polytetrafluoroethylene (PTFE)-covered stents have demonstrated fewer problems with occlusion.[63,64] The other main morbidity of TIPS is associated with the nature of TIPS being a nonselective shunt, and so diverting blood flow away from the liver and into the systemic circulation. This leads to increased risk of developing or exacerbating hepatic encephalopathy.[65] TIPS is currently considered an experimental therapy for well-compensated patients with HRS who do not respond to medical treatment.[66] The American Association for the Study of Liver Diseases does not recommend TIPS for the treatment of HRS pending the publication of controlled trials; however, the IAC comments that it is a viable option for HRS in patients with a CTP score of 11 or less and serum bilirubin of 5 mg/dL or less.[5,63]

Renal Replacement Therapy

Renal replacement therapy (RRT) is, like other therapies, mostly a consideration for patients who are candidates for liver transplantation. In patients who are not candidates, the risks of the morbidity and mortality that accompany RRT outweigh the benefits because of the dismal likelihood of survival without a transplant. Although establishment of chronic hemodialysis (HD) in these patients can prolong survival, 33% of the days of life gained are spent in the hospital because of the high rates of morbidity caused by HD.[67]

As a bridge to transplant (BTT), RRT is a reasonable option for patients who failed other therapies for HRS and have indications for RRT, such as progressing metabolic acidosis, hyperkalemia, and volume overload. The most efficacious type of RRT has not been revealed; however, this is typically governed by the clinical status of the patient. The use of continuous renal replacement therapy (CRRT) has benefits over intermittent HD in patients with hepatic failure because of its ability to improve cardiovascular stability and to cause less fluctuation in intracranial pressure.[68,69] It also has the theoretical advantage of removing inflammatory cytokines.[70,71] Despite these theoretical advantages, clinical studies have mostly shown the opposite. Patients receiving CRRT have had higher mortality rates in clinical trials than those receiving intermittent HD; however, this is most likely because of the severity of illness and unstable clinical condition present.[72] In one large analysis, for example, patients with cirrhosis who received CRRT had a 73% mortality rate compared with 50% in patients who received HD. It is important to note, however, that a large percentage of the patients survived to transplantation (26% and 42%, respectively).[73] From the data available, it appears that either HD or CRRT may be used before transplantation, and the modality of RRT should be governed by the patient's clinical status.

The molecular adsorbent recirculating system (MARS) is a modified dialysis method that uses an albumin-containing dialysate allowing for the selective removal of albumin-bound substances. It is recirculated and recycled within the system using charcoal and anion-exchanger columns. It was originally used as a "liver dialysis" that prolonged survival in patients with fulminant hepatic failure and acute-on-chronic hepatic failure as a BTT. With the observation that MARS had a good clinical impact on patients with HRS, 2 centers performed a randomized, controlled trial comparing it to standard care. They used an especially high-risk patient population with bilirubin concentrations of 15 mg/dL or higher and CTP scores higher than 12, a group that is contraindicated against a TIPS procedure. With only 13 patients, they were still able to show that the use of MARS improved survival rates at day 7 compared with the control group (37.5% vs 0%) and 25% of patients on MARS were still alive at day 30. This is a significant finding in a severely critically ill population.[74] The same group also demonstrated that MARS showed significant improvement in other organs in patients with HRS in addition to the renal function.[75] These successes have prompted the attempt to use MARS in patients who have failed standard vasoconstrictor therapy with octreotide and midodrine, which was met with poor results in an analysis of 6 patients. MARS did not improve systemic or renal hemodynamics or improve renal function in this critically ill population.[76]

Liver Transplantation

Liver transplantation remains the treatment of choice for patients with type 1 HRS because it allows for both the liver disease and associated renal failure to be cured. The most current Scientific Registry of Transplant Recipients (SRTR) data analysis shows that deceased donor liver transplant recipients are achieving 87% survival at 1 year and 73% at 5 years, which is much better than any other management of HRS.[77] After liver transplantation, the systemic hemodynamic abnormalities return to near-normal at 2 weeks posttransplant and completely normalize within 2 months.[78] Before the adoption of the model for end-stage liver disease (MELD) score for the allocation of liver transplants in the United States in 2002, patients largely received transplants based on their time on the waiting list and CTP score, which did not take into account renal function.[79] This put patients with type 1 HRS at a significant disadvantage. The current allocation based on severity of liver disease with the MELD system is more objective and improves the chances of patients with HRS receiving a liver transplant before death. However, the MELD score was validated as a predictor of 90-day survival in patients with chronic liver disease and not HRS. In a recent analysis of 105 patients with HRS, it was found that patients with type 1 HRS had a significantly higher mortality rate than was predicted using the MELD score.[80] This study demonstrates that it may be necessary to have an "exception" for patients with type 1 HRS to increase their MELD score, similar to what is currently in use for patients with hepatocellular carcinoma (HCC) who meet the Milan criteria.

It has been demonstrated that pretransplant renal function predicts morbidity and mortality posttransplant, including longer ICU stays, higher incidence of need for dialysis, and higher mortality at 30 days and 2 years.[81,82] Specifically, patients with HRS had longer stays in the ICU and required more dialysis treatments compared with those patients without HRS who received transplants, although they had similar 2-year graft survival.[83] It is important to point out that this analysis used an outdated definition for HRS and did not differentiate between types 1 and 2 HRS. In a more recent study, however, patients with HRS who were treated with vasopressin analogs had similar 3-year mortality rates (83% vs 100%), days in the ICU, and infections compared with patients without HRS who received transplants.[41] A larger analysis with longer follow-up is necessary to determine whether pretransplant treatment of HRS would have an impact on posttransplant outcomes.[6]

The reported rate of renal recovery after transplantation has varied in many analyses. Although Gonwa and colleagues[83] demonstrated that only 10% of patients with HRS developed end-stage renal disease after transplantation, this was, again, using an outdated definition of HRS and did not differentiate between type 1 or 2. Conversely in a more recent analysis of exclusively patients with type 1 HRS, 58% of patients remained dialysis dependent after liver transplantation.[84] Reversal of renal dysfunction may be more likely in patients who have had renal dysfunction for shorter durations of time. It has been shown that, regardless of diagnosis of HRS or not, patients with an SrCr of 1.5 mg/dL or higher for more than 3.6 weeks were significantly less likely to recover renal function.[85] A study to ascertain what circumstances would make combined liver-kidney transplantation (CLKT) beneficial found a survival advantage in patients who were on pretransplant HD for more than 8 weeks.[86] Schmitt and colleagues,[87] analyzing the United Network for Organ Sharing (UNOS) database, found that patients who undergo CLKT who are on HD before transplantation had a 1-year survival advantage compared with patients with an SrCr of 2.5 mg/dL or higher who were not on dialysis, indicating that dialysis-dependent patients are best benefited. In support, the most recent SRTR report shows that patients who were on HD at the time of transplant had 2-year survival advantage (75.9% vs 70.8%) if they received a CLKT instead of a liver transplant alone.[88] These data are limited by many shortcomings that are seen in retrospective single-center and database analyses, however, demonstrating the difficulty in deciding on the duration of renal dysfunction for candidacy for CLKT. At the Consensus Conference for Simultaneous Liver Kidney Transplant in 2008, experts recommended that the only patients with HRS who would be considered candidates for CKLT are patients who have had an SrCr of 2 mg/dL or higher and dialysis for 8 weeks or longer.[88]

SUMMARY

The past 5 decades have cast light on much of the epidemiology of HRS. Many therapies for managing HRS have been found that can be effective, although all have downsides and are predominantly bridges to transplant. Because of the extremely poor prognosis, much effort is being put toward improving management of this syndrome. Studies to better delineate which therapies best improve chances of renal recovery after transplant and what patients are best served by CLKT are eagerly awaited.

ACKNOWLEDGMENTS

Special acknowledgment to Anita Patel, MD, Transplant Nephrologist, Division of Transplant, Henry Ford Hospital, Detroit, MI, for her expert review and guidance.

REFERENCES

1. Hecker R, Sherlock S. Electrolyte and circulatory changes in terminal liver failure. Lancet 1956;271:1121–5.
2. Koppel MH, Coburn JW, Mims MM, et al. Transplantation of cadaveric kidneys from patients with hepatorenal syndrome. Evidence for the functional nature of renal failure in advanced liver disease. N Engl J Med 1969;280(25):1367–71.
3. Iwatsuki S, Popovtzer MM, Corman JL, et al. Recovery from "hepatorenal syndrome" after orthotopic liver transplantation. N Engl J Med 1973;289(22):1155–9.
4. Arroyo V, Gines P, Gerbes A, et al. Definition and diagnostic criteria of refractory ascites and hepatorenal syndrome in cirrhosis. Hepatology 1996;23(1):164–76.
5. Salerno F, Gerbes A, Gines P, et al. Diagnosis, prevention, and treatment of hepatorenal syndrome in cirrhosis. Postgrad Med J 2008;84:662–70.
6. Wadei HM, Mai ML, Ahsan N, et al. Hepatorenal syndrome: pathophysiology and management. Clin J Am Soc Nephrol 2006;1:1066–79.
7. Tristani FE, Cohn JN. Systemic and renal hemodynamics in oliguric hepatic failure: effect of volume expansion. J Clin Invest 1967;46(12):1894–906.
8. Ruiz-del-Arbol L, Urman J, Fernandez J, et al. Systemic, renal, and hepatic hemodynamic derangement in cirrhotic patients with spontaneous bacterial peritonitis. Hepatology 2003;38(5):1210–8.
9. Ruiz-del-Arbol L, Monescillo A, Arocena C, et al. Circulatory function and hepatorenal syndrome in cirrhosis. Hepatology 2005;42:439–47.
10. Schroeder ET, Eich RH, Smulyan H, et al. Plasma renin levels in hepatic cirrhosis. Relationship to functional renal failure. Am J Med 1970;49:186–91.
11. Henriksen JH, Ring-Larsen H. Hepatorenal disorders: role of the sympathetic nervous system. Semin Liver Dis 1994;14(1):35–43.
12. Boyer TD, Zia P, Reynolds TB. Effects of indomethacin and prostaglandin A1 in renal function and plasma renin activity in alcoholic liver disease. Gastroenterology 1979;77:215–22.
13. Schrier RW, Arroyo V, Bernardi M, et al. Peripheral arterial vasodilation hypothesis: a proposal for the initiation of renal sodium and retention in cirrhosis. Hepatology 1988;8(5):1151–7.
14. Iwao T, Oho K, Sakai T, et al. Splanchnic and extrasplanchnic arterial hemodynamics in patients with cirrhosis. J Hepatol 1997;27:817–23.
15. Solis-Herruzo JA, Duran A, Favela V, et al. Effects of lumbar sympathetic block on kidney function in cirrhotic patients with hepatorenal syndrome. J Hepatol 1987;5:167–73.
16. Torregrosa M, Aguade S, Dos L, et al. Cardiac alterations in cirrhosis: reversibility after liver transplantation. J Hepatol 2005;42:68–74.
17. Sort P, Navasa M, Arroyo V, et al. Effect of intravenous albumin on renal impairment and mortality in patients with cirrhosis and spontaneous bacterial peritonitis. N Engl J Med 1999;341(6):403–9.
18. Lluch P, Mauricio MD, Vila JM, et al. Accumulation of symmetric dimethylarginine in hepatorenal syndrome. Exp Biol Med (Maywood) 2006;231(1):70–5.
19. Gines A, Escorsell A, Gines P, et al. Incidence, predictive factors, and prognosis of the hepatorenal syndrome in cirrhosis with ascites. Gastroenterology 1993;105:229–36.
20. Fernandez J, Navasa M, Planas R, et al. Primary prophylaxis of spontaneous bacterial peritonitis delays hepatorenal syndrome and improves survival in cirrhosis. Gastroenterology 2007;133:818–24.

21. Planas R, Montoliu S, Balleste B, et al. Natural history of patients hospitalized for management of cirrhotic ascites. Clin Gastroenterol Hepatol 2006;4:1385–94.
22. Follo A, Llovet JM, Navasa M, et al. Renal impairment after spontaneous bacterial peritonitis in cirrhosis: incidence, clinical course, predictive factors, and prognosis. Hepatology 1994;20(6):1495–501.
23. Gines P, Tito L, Arroyo V, et al. Randomized comparative study of therapeutic paracentesis with and without intravenous albumin in cirrhosis. Gastroenterology 1988;94:1493–502.
24. Cardenas A, Gines P, Uriz J, et al. Renal failure after upper GI bleeding in cirrhosis: incidence, clinical course, predictive factors, and short-term prognosis. Hepatology 2001;34(4):671–6.
25. Cabrera J, Arroyo V, Ballesta AM, et al. Aminoglycoside nephrotoxicity in cirrhosis: value of urinary β_2-microglobulin to discriminate functional renal failure from acute tubular damage. Gastroenterology 1982;82:97–105.
26. Moore KP, Wong F, Gines P, et al. The management of ascites in cirrhosis: report on the Consensus Conference of the International Ascites Club. Hepatology 2003;38(1):258–66.
27. Garcia-Compean D, Blanc P, Larrey D, et al. Treatment of cirrhotic tense ascites with dextran-40 versus albumin associated with large volume paracentesis: a randomized controlled trial. Ann Hepatol 2002;1(1):29–35.
28. Lin SM, Lee CS, Kao PF. Low-dose dopamine infusion in cirrhosis with refractory ascites. Int J Clin Pract 1998;52:533–6.
29. Vincenti F, Goldberg LI. Combined use of dopamine and prostaglandin A1 in patients with acute renal failure and hepatorenal syndrome. Prostaglandins 1978;15(3):463–72.
30. Durkin RJ, Winter SM. Reversal of hepatorenal syndrome with the combination of norepinephrine and dopamine. Crit Care Med 1995;23(1):202–4.
31. Gulberg V, Bilzer M, Gerbes AL. Long-term therapy and retreatment of hepatorenal syndrome type 1 with ornipressin and dopamine. Hepatology 1999;30:870–5.
32. Guevara M, Gines P, Fernandez-Esparrach G, et al. Reversibility of hepatorenal syndrome by prolonged administration of ornipressin and plasma volume expansion. Hepatology 1998;27:35–41.
33. Lenz K, Hortnagl H, Druml W, et al. Beneficial effect of 8-ornithin vasopressin on renal dysfunction in decompensated cirrhosis. Gut 1989;30:90–6.
34. Presurato AB, Jennings HR, Voils SA. Terlipressin: vasopressin analogue and novel drug for septic shock. Ann Pharmacother 2006;40:2170–7.
35. Sanyal AJ, Boyer T, Garcia-Tsao G, et al. A randomized, prospective, double-blind, placebo-controlled trial of terlipressin for type 1 hepatorenal syndrome. Gastroenterology 2008;134:1360–8.
36. Colle I, Durand F, Pessione F, et al. Clinical course, predictive factors and prognosis in patients with cirrhosis and type 1 hepatorenal syndrome treated with terlipressin: a retrospective analysis. J Gastroenterol Hepatol 2002;17:882–8.
37. Uriz J, Gines P, Cardenas A, et al. Terlipressin plus albumin infusion: an effective and safe therapy of hepatorenal syndrome. J Hepatol 2000;33:43–8.
38. Solanki P, Chawla A, Garg R, et al. Beneficial effects of terlipressin in hepatorenal syndrome: a prospective, randomized, placebo-controlled clinical trial. J Gastroenterol Hepatol 2003;18:152–6.
39. Ortega R, Gines P, Uriz J, et al. Terlipressin therapy with and without albumin for patients with hepatorenal syndrome: results of a prospective, nonrandomized study. Hepatology 2002;36(4):941–8.

40. Martin-Llahi M, Pepin M, Guevara M, et al. Terlipressin and albumin vs. albumin in patients with cirrhosis and hepatorenal syndrome: a randomized study. Gastroenterology 2008;134:1352–9.
41. Restuccia T, Ortega R, Guevara M, et al. Effects of treatment of hepatorenal syndrome before transplantation on posttransplantation outcome. A case control study. J Hepatol 2004;40:140–6.
42. Angeli P, Volpin R, Gerunda G, et al. Reversal of type 1 hepatorenal syndrome with the administration of midodrine and octreotide. Hepatology 1999;29(6): 1690–7.
43. Seiber CC, Lee FY, Groszmann RJ. Long-term octreotide treatment prevents vascular hyporeactivity in portal-hypertensive rats. Hepatology 1996;23: 1218–23.
44. Esrailian E, Pantangco E, Kyulo N, et al. Octreotide/midodrine therapy significantly improves renal function and 30-day survival in patients with type 1 hepatorenal syndrome. Dig Dis Sci 2007;52:742–8.
45. Kiser TH, Fish DN, Obritsch MD, et al. Vasopressin, not octreotide, may be beneficial in the treatment of hepatorenal syndrome: a retrospective study. Nephrol Dial Transplant 2005;20:1813–20.
46. Obritsch MD, Jung R, Fish DN, et al. Effects of continuous vasopressin infusion in patients with septic shock. Ann Pharmacother 2004;38:1117–22.
47. Duvoux C, Zanditenas D, Hezode C, et al. Effects of noradrenalin and albumin in patients with type 1 HRS: a pilot study. Hepatology 2002;36:374–80.
48. Alessandria C, Ottobrelli A, Debernardi-Vernon W, et al. Noradrenalin vs terlipressin in patient with hepatorenal syndrome: a prospective, randomized, unblinded, pilot study. J Hepatol 2007;47:499–505.
49. Sharma P, Kumar A, Sharma B, et al. An open label, pilot, randomized controlled trial of noradrenalin versus terlipressin in the treatment of type 1 hepatorenal syndrome and predictors of response. Am J Gastroenterol 2008;103:1689–97.
50. Boyer TD. Transjugular intrahepatic portosystemic shunt: current status. Gastroenterology 2003;124:1700–10.
51. Shiffman ML, Jeffers L, Hoofnagle JH, et al. The role of transjugular intrahepatic portosystemic shunt for treatment of portal hypertension and its complications: a conference sponsored by the National Digestive Disease Advisory Board. Hepatology 1995;25:1591–7.
52. Ring EJ, Lake JR, Roberts JP, et al. Using transjugular intrahepatic portosystemic shunt to control variceal bleeding before liver transplantation. Ann Intern Med 1992;116:304–9.
53. Cabrera J, Maynar M, Granados R, et al. Transjugular intrahepatic portosystemic shunt (TIPS) vs. esclerotherapy in the elective treatment of variceal haemorrhage. Gastroenterology 1996;110:832–9.
54. Senzolo M, Cholongitas E, Tibballs J, et al. Transjugular intrahepatic portosystemic shunt in the management of ascites and hepatorenal syndrome. Eur J Gastroenterol Hepatol 2006;18:1143–50.
55. Somberg K, Lake JR, Tomlanovich SJ, et al. Transjugular intrahepatic portosystemic shunts for refractory ascites: assessment of clinical and hormonal response and renal function. Hepatology 1995;21:709.
56. Ochs A, Rossle M, Haag K, et al. The transjugular intrahepatic portosystemic stent-shunt procedure for refractory ascites. N Engl J Med 1995;332:1192.
57. Wong F, Sniderman K, Liu P, et al. Transjugular intrahepatic portosystemic stent shunt: effects on hemodynamics and sodium homeostasis in cirrhosis and refractory ascites. Ann Intern Med 1995;122:816–22.

58. Alam I, Bass NM, LaBerge JM, et al. Treatment of hepatorenal syndrome with the transjugular intrahepatic portosystemic shunt (TIPS). Gastroenterology 1995;108: 1024A.

59. Spahr L, Fenyeves D, N'Guyen VV, et al. Improvement of hepatorenal syndrome by transjugular intrahepatic portosystemic shunt. Am J Gastroenterol 1995;90: 1169–70.

60. Sturgis TM. Hepatorenal syndrome: resolution after transjugular intrahepatic portosystemic shunt. J Clin Gastroenterol 1995;20:241–3.

61. Guevara M, Gines P, Bandi JC, et al. Transjugular intrahepatic portosystemic shunt in hepatorenal syndrome: effects on renal function and vasoactive systems. Hepatology 1998;28:416.

62. Brensing KA, Textor J, Strunk H, et al. Transjugular intrahepatic portosystemic stent-shunt for hepatorenal syndrome [letter]. Lancet 1997;349:697.

63. Boyer TD, Haskal ZJ. The role of transjugular intrahepatic portosystemic shunt in the management of portal hypertension. Hepatology 2005;41:386–400.

64. Bureau C, Garcia-Pagan JC, Otal P, et al. Improved clinical outcome using polytetrafluoroethylene-coated stents for TIPS: results of a randomized study. Gastroenterology 2004;126:469–75.

65. LaBerge JM. Transjugular intrahepatic portosystemic shunt: role in treating intractable variceal bleeding, ascites, and hepatic hydrothorax. Clin Liver Dis 2006;10: 583–98.

66. Munoz SJ. The hepatorenal syndrome. Med Clin North Am 2008;92:813–37.

67. Capling RK, Bastani B. The clinical course of patients with type 1 hepatorenal syndrome maintained on hemodialysis. Ren Fail 2004;26:563–8.

68. Davenport A, Will EJ, Davidson AM. Improved cardiovascular stability during continuous modes of renal replacement therapy in critically ill patients with acute hepatic and renal failure. Crit Care Med 1993;21:328–38.

69. Davenport A. The management of renal failure in patients at risk of cerebral edema/hypoxia. New Horiz 1995;3(4):717–24.

70. Hirasawa H, Oda S, Matsuda K. Continuous hemodiafiltration with cytokine-adsorbing hemofilter in the treatment of severe sepsis and septic shock. Contrib Nephrol 2007;156:365–70.

71. Navasa M, Follo A, Filella X, et al. Tumor necrosis factor and interleukin-6 in spontaneous bacterial peritonitis in cirrhosis: relationship with the development of renal impairment and mortality. Hepatology 1998;27:1227–32.

72. Witzke O, Baumann M, Patschan D, et al. Which patients benefit from hemodialysis therapy in hepatorenal syndrome? J Gastroenterol Hepatol 2004;19(12):1369–73.

73. Wong LP, Blackley MP, Andreoni KA, et al. Survival of liver transplant candidates with acute renal failure receiving renal replacement therapy. Kidney Int 2005;68: 362–70.

74. Mitzner SR, Stange J, Klammt S, et al. Improvement of hepatorenal syndrome with extracorporeal albumin dialysis MARS: results of a prospective, randomized, controlled clinical trial. Liver Transpl 2000;6(3):277–86.

75. Mitzner SR, Klammt S, Peszynski P, et al. Improvement of multiple organ functions in hepatorenal syndrome during albumin dialysis with the molecular adsorbent recirculating system. Ther Apher 2001;5(5):417–22.

76. Wong F, Raina N, Richardson R. Molecular adsorbent recirculating system is ineffective in the management of type 1 hepatorenal syndrome in cirrhotic patients with ascites who have failed vasoconstrictor therapy. Gut 2009;59:381–6.

77. Berg CL, Steffick DE, Edwards EB, et al. Liver and intestine transplantation in the United States 1998–2007. Am J Transplant 2009;9(2):907–31.

78. Navasa M, Feu F, Garcia-Pagan JC, et al. Hemodynamic and humoral changes after liver transplantation in patients with cirrhosis. Hepatology 1993;17(3): 355–60.
79. Weisner R, Edwards E, Freeman R, et al. Model for end-stage liver disease (MELD) and allocation of donor livers. Gastroenterology 2003;124:91–6.
80. Alessandria C, Ozdogan O, Guevara M, et al. MELD score and clinical type predict prognosis in hepatorenal syndrome: relevance to liver transplantation. Hepatology 2005;41(6):1282–9.
81. Lafayette RA, Pare G, Schmid CH, et al. Pretransplant renal dysfunction predicts poorer outcome in liver transplantation. Clin Nephrol 1997;49(3):159–64.
82. Nair S, Verma S, Thulavath PJ. Pretransplant renal function predicts survival in patients undergoing orthotopic liver transplantation. Hepatology 2002;35: 1179–85.
83. Gonwa TA, Morris CA, Goldstein RM, et al. Long-term survival and renal function following liver transplantation in patients with and without hepatorenal syndrome—experience in 300 patients. Transplantation 1991;51(2):428–30.
84. Marik PE, Wood K, Starzl TE. The course of type 1 hepatorenal syndrome post liver transplantation. Nephrol Dial Transplant 2006;21:478–82.
85. Campbell MS, Kotlyar DS, Brensinger CM, et al. Renal function after orthotopic liver transplantation is predicted by duration of pretransplantation creatinine elevation. Liver Transpl 2005;11(9):1048–55.
86. Ruiz R, Kunitake H, Wilkinson AH, et al. Long-term analysis of combined liver and kidney transplantation at a single center. Arch Surg 2006;141:735–41.
87. Schmitt TM, Kumer SC, Al-Osaimi A, et al. Combined liver-kidney and liver transplantation in patients with renal failure outcomes in the MELD-era. Transpl Int 2009;22:876–83.
88. Eason JD, Gonwa TA, Davis CL, et al. Proceedings of consensus conference on simultaneous liver kidney transplantation (SLK). Am J Transplant 2008;8: 2243–51.

Nutrition Support in End-Stage Liver Disease

Vivian M. Zhao, PharmD, BCNSP[a],*, Thomas R. Ziegler, MD[b,c,d]

KEYWORDS

• Amino acids • Liver failure • End-stage liver disease
• Malnutrition • Nutrition support

Protein-calorie malnutrition (PCM) results after several weeks to months of insufficient dietary intake of protein and calories, increased protein and energy requirements, impaired use of macronutrients (eg, protein, carbohydrates, lipid, and total energy), or malabsorption of protein and energy, respectively. PCM is an increasingly recognized complication in both alcoholic and nonalcoholic liver disease.[1–5] PCM is associated with increased morbidity and mortality[2,4] in patients with end-stage liver disease (ESLD), including those awaiting liver transplantation.[6–9] The liver facilitates the synthesis of key plasma proteins; plays a major role in regulation of carbohydrate, fat, and protein metabolism; and serves as a major storage site for glycogen, iron, copper, fat soluble vitamins A, D, E, K, and vitamin B_{12}. The liver also plays a central role in the detoxification and excretion of waste productions, including ammonia, bacteria, bilirubin, and medications. Unfortunately, PCM is frequently underdiagnosed in patients with ESLD.[1]

PREVALENCE

PCM is nearly universal in patients with ESLD. The degree of malnutrition is directly correlated with the severity of liver disease irrespective of the cause.[4,9,10] Although PCM is not typically a complication of acute liver disease, it occurs in up to 20% of those with mild or chronic liver disease without cirrhosis.[1,11] The prevalence of

This work was supported by National Institutes of Health grant K24 RR023356 (TRZ).
[a] Nutrition and Metabolic Support Service, Department of Pharmaceutical Services, Emory University Hospital, 1364 Clifton Road, NE, Atlanta, GA 30322, USA
[b] Nutrition and Metabolic Support Service, Emory University Hospital, 1364 Clifton Road, NE, Atlanta, GA 30322, USA
[c] Division of Endocrinology, Metabolism and Lipids, Department of Medicine, Emory University School of Medicine, Suite GC-23, 1364 Clifton Road, NE, Atlanta, GA, USA
[d] Atlanta Clinical & Translational Science Institute, Emory University Hospital, Suite GG-23, 1364 Clifton Road, Atlanta, GA 30322, USA
* Corresponding author.
E-mail address: vivian.zhao@emoryhealthcare.org

Crit Care Nurs Clin N Am 22 (2010) 369–380
doi:10.1016/j.ccell.2010.02.003
0899-5885/10/$ – see front matter. Published by Elsevier Inc.
ccnursing.theclinics.com

malnutrition is as high as 65% to 90% of those with advanced liver disease[1-4] and nearly 100% of liver transplant candidates.[12] PCM occurs with roughly equal incidence in both nonalcoholic and alcoholic cirrhosis.[4,5] In addition, a variety of micronutrient and vitamin deficiencies are frequently seen in patients with ESLD.[13-15] Patients with cholestasis are at much higher risk to develop fat-soluble vitamin deficiencies than liver disease patients without cholestasis.[16,17]

MECHANISMS OF MALNUTRITION

Hepatic function is often well preserved into the late stages of the liver disease process; approximately 90% of hepatic cells are injured before nutrition-related functions are impaired.[18] Development of malnutrition in patients with ESLD is multifactorial, but three major factors appear to play a major role: poor dietary intake, impaired nutrients digestion or absorption, and altered nutrient metabolism. The underlying mechanisms of these are not well understood, yet each appears to worsen with the progression of liver disease.

Poor Dietary Intake

A primary cause of malnutrition in liver failure is poor dietary intake, which may stem from several factors. Patients with chronic liver disease often exhibit nausea, anorexia, and altered taste sensation, which may decrease overall food intake. Poor intake has been associated with various nutrient deficiencies and is associated with an increase in tissue and plasma levels of proinflammatory cytokines such as tumor necrosis factor alpha.[19,20] Furthermore, altered mental status due to hepatic encephalopathy can contribute to diminished overall dietary intake. In addition, early satiety may result from the presence of ascites or increased blood leptin level in ESLD.[21] Restrictive diets are commonly prescribed to patients with ESLD, including those with restrictions of dietary sodium, protein, or fluid, and may lead to inadequate oral intake. In patients who have fully recovered from adequately treated hepatic encephalopathy, inappropriate long-term protein restriction may further aggravate protein losses.

Malabsorption

Malabsorption is another important contributor to malnutrition in patients with ESLD. Malabsorption of nutrients varies considerably among this patient population, and a variety of mechanisms may contribute to poor nutrient absorption. In cholestatic patients, reduced intraluminal bile-salt secretion and pool size may lead to steatorrhea. Fat malabsorption from the gastrointestinal tract contributes to energy depletion and deficiencies in fat-soluble vitamins (vitamins A, D, E, and K). Concomitant conditions such as small intestinal mucosal disease (eg, inflammatory bowel disease, celiac sprue) or pancreatic insufficiency may further hinder the digestion and absorption of nutrients if these conditions remain undetected. The presence of bacteria overgrowth resulting from impaired small bowel motility has also been implicated as a cause of malabsorption in ESLD.[22] Another potential mechanism that contributes to poor absorption is portal hypertension in patients with advanced liver failure.[23] In addition, the administration of commonly prescribed medications, such as neomycin, cholestyramine, and lactulose, may adversely affect nutrient absorption.

Metabolic Abnormalities

An important cause of PCM in patients with advanced liver disease is serious metabolic abnormalities (**Box 1**). In patients with ESLD, there is a more rapid transition from the use of carbohydrates to the use of fat stores as a substrate for metabolism, which is

---

Box 1
Abnormal fuel metabolism observed in liver failure

Carbohydrate

- Increased glucose intolerance
- Increased insulin resistance
- Increased gluconeogenesis
- Decreased glycogen synthesis

Protein or Amino Acids

- Increased rate of protein catabolism
- Decreased rate of protein synthesis
- Increased peripheral use of branched-chain amino acids (BCAAs)
- Increased ureagenesis
- Erosion of lean body mass and negative nitrogen balance

Fat

- Increased lipolysis
- Increased oxidation of nonesterified fatty acids
- Increased ketogenesis

---

similar to the metabolic impairments that mimic a hypercatabolic state in a healthy subject after 72 hours of starvation.[24,25] This is presumably a response to the decreases in both carbohydrate use and hepatic glycogen storage that is observed in patients with ESLD. Insulin resistance and impaired glycogen storage lead to a greater dependence and earlier use of fat and protein as a fuel source. This, in turn, leads to depletion of fat and protein reserves in the settings of inadequate nutrient intake. Increased peripheral lipolysis that occurs in ESLD may also lead to increased free fatty acid (FFA) turnover or oxidation and ketone body production.[26] The elevated FFA levels may further aggravate insulin resistance. In addition, the storage of fatty acid in the form of triglycerides may be impaired owing to inhibition of lipoprotein lipase and decreased availability of glycerol as a contributor to gluconeogenesis.

Protein metabolism is also altered in patients with ESLD, with net protein break-down being common. After an overnight fast, there is an early switch to gluconeogenesis from amino acids by mobilizing amino acids from the skeletal muscle because of insufficient hepatic glycogen reserves and impaired synthetic capacity of the hepatic cell.[24,25] It has been observed that among cirrhotic patients, the plasma levels of branched-chain amino acids (ie, leucine, isoleucine, and valine) are reduced, whereas the levels of aromatic amino acids (ie, phenylalanine, tyrosine, and tryptophan) are elevated because of the dependence of hepatic metabolic pathways.[27]

Hypermetabolism as a contributor to malnutrition continues to be debated by investigators. It is unclear whether the increased energy expenditure seen in some patients is induced by hepatic dysfunction or its associated complications.[8,28] Up to one-third of patients with cirrhosis are considered hypermetabolic[29] with resting energy expenditures of 120% of the expected value.[30] There is a great variability in energy expenditure in this patient population; up to one-third of patients with cirrhosis have been found to be hypometabolic.[29] Although the exact cause of hypermetabolism remains unclear, there are predisposing factors, such as infection, ascites, and altered patterns of fuel metabolism.[26,31] The use of indirect calorimetry is required to diagnose hypermetabolism; however, this is a not practical approach in daily practice owing to limited accessibility of indirect calorimetry to most clinicians.

ASSESSMENT OF MALNUTRITION

In light of the disturbances in energy production and use and nutrient metabolism in ESLD, it is essential to assess the nutritional status for every patient with chronic liver disease and identify those at risk of developing preventable complications.[32] A comprehensive nutrition assessment consists of four main components: historical background, physical examination, biochemical analysis, and anthropometric studies (**Box 2**). This, however, is not always easily accomplished. The manifestations of malnourishment can vary considerably between patients, even in those with the same cause and severity of illness. Parameters commonly used for nutritional assessment, such as body weight changes, are influenced by liver disease and its related complications (eg, fluid retention). There are no consensuses on assessment parameters that are diagnostic for malnutrition per se in patients with chronic liver disease.

Biochemical Nutritional Markers

The conventional blood tests traditionally used as protein biomarkers are poor predictors to detect PCM in ESLD. In general, serum albumin is not a good measure of protein status because of its relatively long half-life (18 to 21 days) and that serum concentrations can be affected by nonnutritional factors (anabolic steroids and exogenous albumin). Serum proteins with shorter half-lives including transferrin, retinol-binding protein, and prealbumin more accurately reflect protein status. These biochemical markers are generally unreliable because of impaired hepatic protein synthesis in correlation with the severity of liver dysfunction rather than poor nutritional status.[33] In addition, serum protein status is susceptible to alterations in fluid status, micronutrient status, and renal function. In ESLD patients, circulating concentrations of proteins (eg, albumin, prealbumin), are often decreased owing to inflammation or infection, or fluid overload and are not useful as protein nutrition biomarkers given their lack of specificity. Malnutrition can reduce immune function. Immunologic parameters, such as total lymphocyte count and delayed hypersensitivity skin reactions, are abnormal in cirrhotic patients, and the abnormalities can occur independent of nutritional status.[34] Therefore, consideration must be given to the patient's clinical state when interpreting laboratory measurements used in nutrition assessment.

Anthropometric Parameters

Simple anthropometric parameters used to reflect body composition includes weight, height, midarm muscle circumference (MAMC), and triceps skin-fold thickness (TSF). Body weight is an insensitive and unreliable indicator in the presence of ascites and edema. In turn, malnourishment might actually be hidden by fluid gains. MAMC and TSF assess skeletal muscle mass and fat storage, respectively. They are reasonably accurate even in the presence of fluid retention because edema accumulates to a lesser extent in the upper extremities. MAMC has been shown to be an independent predictor of mortality[6,35] and has demonstrated prognostic significance when combined with the Child-Turcotte-Pugh scores.[6] The lack of calibrated equipment, as well as intra- and interobserver error, limits the validity and reproducibility of these interpretations.[10] Alternatively, assessment of muscle function, such as hand-grip strength and respiratory-muscle strength have also been used in nutritional evaluation. However, these measurements tend to be more useful in monitoring changes in patient's status over time.[34]

Box 2
Nutritional assessment and treatment in patients with ESLD

1. Review medical and surgical history (both acute and chronic)

   - Presence of concomitant conditions (eg, small intestine diseases, renal failure, pancreatic insufficiency)

   - Degree of liver failure (eg, cirrhosis, encephalopathy, liver transplantation candidate)

   - Use of medications that may decrease nutrient absorption (eg, neomycin, cholestyramine, lactulose), increase nutrient excretion (eg, loop diuretics)

2. Perform subjective global assessment

   - Signs of muscle or fat wasting, micronutrient deficiencies (eg, night blindness, altered taste)

   - Presence of edema or ascites

   - Gastrointestinal (GI) related symptoms (eg, nausea, vomiting, diarrhea, GI bleeding)

   - Obtain actual body weight (dry weight; patients without ascites or edema) or calculate ideal body weight (patients with ascites or edema); determine percent weight loss during the previous 6 months

   - Assess functional status that may impair dietary intake (eg, altered mental status, decreased functional capacity)

   - Evaluate changes in dietary intake including general food and beverage consumption patterns, use of vitamins and mineral supplementations

3. Obtain biochemical measurements

   - Organ function indices, electrolytes, and selected vitamin and mineral concentration as indicated by medical history, subjective global assessment, or underlying diseases

4. Determine caloric (kcal) and protein needs: 25–35 kcal/kg/d and 1.2–1.5 g/kg/d protein (use actual or ideal body weight dependent of the presence of ascites or edema)

5. Implement appropriate nutritional support

   - Optimize oral intake

     4 to 7 meals per day includes a late evening or bedtime carbohydrate-rich snacks

     Dietary restriction (eg, restrict fluid if sodium <120 mEq; restrict sodium if ascites or edema is present)

     Consider oral supplementation if general food intake is inadequate

   - Maximize hepatic encephalopathy treatment

     Optimize medication treatment, treat underlying disease

     Restrict protein only if protein intolerance and keep restriction as brief as possible

     Consider BCAAs-supplemented nutrition in encephalopathy III or IV

   - Consider enteral and parenteral nutrition (PN) when dietary modifications or enteral tube feeding fail to maintain nutritional status, respectively

   - Provide multivitamins and correct specific vitamins and mineral deficiency

---

Bioelectrical impedance analysis (BIA) is a reliable and more readily available tool for many patient populations. Unfortunately, it has been shown to be unreliable in cirrhotic patients with fluid disturbances.[36,37] Other sophisticated techniques used to measure body cell mass are in vivo neutron activation analysis (IVNAA), dual energy X-ray absorptiometry (DEXA), and isotope dilution. Currently, these techniques are employed as research tools only.[11]

Subjective Global Assessment

Subjective global assessment (SGA) is recommended by the European Society for Clinical Nutrition and Metabolism (ESPEN) as a practical bedside method in assessing malnourished patients.[32,34] It combines multiple nutritional assessment components, including weight loss during the previous 6 months, changes in dietary intake, decreased functional capacity, physical examination (muscle wasting, loss of subcutaneous fat, edema, or ascites), underlying disease, and gastrointestinal symptoms (diarrhea, nausea, and vomiting) that have persisted for greater than 2 weeks, to classify the severity of malnutrition. Some studies have found it to be imprecise, with a high specificity but a poor sensitivity, especially in alcoholic cirrhosis.[38]

NUTRITIONAL THERAPY

In light of the high incidence of malnutrition among patients with ESLD, the ultimate goal of nutritional therapy is to maintain or replete muscle and fat stores. The first line of nutritional intervention is optimizing the oral intake. If dietary intake is insufficient to maintain desired nutritional status, then oral supplementations, enteral nutrition, parenteral nutrition (PN), or a combination should be used to correct nutritional deficiencies.

Energy and Protein Intake

The consensus report by ESPEN on nutrition support in liver disease has recommendations for both caloric and protein intake goals for patients with chronic liver disease.[11,39,40] The most recent consensus reports recommend an intake of 35 to 40 kcal/kg/d[38] or approximately 130% of the measured or estimated resting energy expenditure[40] and 1.2 to 1.5 g/kg/d of protein for all cirrhotic patients.[39,40] When estimating caloric and protein intakes, the actual body weight should be used for cirrhotic patients without ascites, whereas the ideal body weight should be used for patients with ascites.[40] Routine protein restriction in hepatic encephalopathy should be continued as briefly as possible. In fact, Cordoba and colleagues[41] have suggested that normal oral protein intake did not adversely affect clinical outcomes and survival in these patients. Of note, the European clinical practice guidelines suggest that protein intake need not be restricted in patients with ESLD encephalopathy. These recommendations, however, are based upon expert opinion or clinical experience and the unblinded study of enteral diet in non-ICU patients by Cordoba and colleagues.[41] In patients with ESLD and encephalopathy in the ICU, we have adopted the conservative approach of limiting the protein or amino acid dose, at least for several days, to diminish the effect of this potential contributor to mental status changes during diagnostic evaluation.

Dietary Therapy

Dietary therapy is the mainstay for long-term nutritional support in patients with ESLD. A dietary plan that relies minimally on hepatic function while providing adequate protein and calories could reduce the need for supplemental nutrition in this patient population. Dietary restrictions can alleviate some symptoms associated with advanced liver disease. Restriction of sodium is crucial to control ascites and peripheral edema, and it minimizes the need for diuretic therapies. A low sodium diet of 2 to 2.4 g per day or less 200 mg per meal is recommended. Fluid restriction may be implemented in the presence of low serum sodium (<120 mEq/L) and fluid retention.[11] For encephalopathic patients, protein restriction should only be used as last resort when there is no improvement with medication treatments and after correction of any underlying causes (ie, gastrointestinal bleed, infections). Adequate protein intake is required to keep fluid in the arteries and veins rather than leaking into tissue.

The appropriate distribution of caloric intake throughout the day is important to maximize nutrient intake and absorption in this patient population. Several studies have recommended modifying the eating pattern by consuming 4 to 7 small meals daily, including a late evening or bedtime carbohydrate-rich snack.[11,42,43] Eating a late evening snack has been shown to improve nitrogen balance,[42,43] nonprotein respiratory quotient, and protein metabolism,[44] and partially alleviate the abnormal lipid oxidation by reducing the length of overnight fast.[42,43]

Enteral Nutrition

When dietary modifications are insufficient to maintain adequate nutrition intake, enteral nutrition (oral nutritional supplements or tube feeding) should be initiated as soon as possible in this patient population.[39,45] Supplemental enteral nutrition in severely malnourished alcoholic patients with cirrhosis was associated with reduced mortality when compared with patients who received inadequate oral nutrition.[3,43,46,47] Additional benefits of enteral nutrition in these patients included improved Child-Turcotte-Pugh scores, serum albumin levels, bilirubin levels, and hepatic encephalopathy compared with conventional diet.[46–48]

If oral nutritional supplementation is inadequate to meet caloric requirements, enteral tube feeding may be required to ensure adequate nutrient provision. Enteral tube feeding can be safely initiated even in patients with esophageal varices.[39] Tube feeding can be delivered via nasogastric tube (short-term) or percutaneous endoscopic gastrostomy (PEG) tube (long-term). It is important to recognize, however, that PEG tube placement is associated with an increased risk of complications and is contraindicated in cirrhotic patients with ascites, coagulation disorders, interposed organs, peritonitis, and impaired portosystemic collateral circulation secondary to portal hypertension.[39,49] Standard whole protein formulas are preferred for most cirrhotic patients, except for those with fluid retention, in whom a concentrated caloric-dense formula is recommended.[11,39]

PN

PN is reserved for patients who cannot be nourished sufficiently by the mouth or enteral route. Compared with enteral nutrition, PN is a less desirable option because it has not been shown to be more effective at maintaining nutritional status, it is more costly, and it is associated with potential complications, such as bacterial translocation from the gut lumen, which has been associated with increased infection risk.[50] Interestingly, Plauth and colleagues[51] did find that PN might be superior to enteral feeding in patients with transjugular intrahepatic portosystemic shunt, because enteral feeding might worsen hyperammonemia. PN is also indicated in patients with unprotected airway and advanced encephalopathy with compromised cough and swallow reflexes.[40] Of note, PN has been associated with development of increased transaminase levels and hepatic steatosis, especially in patients who are overfed.[52]

Branched-Chain Amino Acid Supplementation

Branched-chain amino acids (BCAA; leucine, isoleucine, and valine) constitute 35% of total muscle protein. The depletion of BCAA, as seen in many cirrhotic patients, might promote the development of hepatic encephalopathy. BCAA depletion enhances the passage of aromatic amino acids (AAA) across the blood-brain barrier and may lead to neurotransmitter synthesis. Therefore, it was hypothesized that BCAA supplementation might improve hepatic encephalopathy by correcting an imbalanced BCAA to

AAA ratio, in which exogenous BCAA compete with AAA for entry across blood brain barrier. In addition, supplementation with BCAA has been shown to inhibit muscle protein breakdown and to increase synthesis of hepatic and muscle protein. Nevertheless, the usefulness of BCAA supplementation in patients with advanced liver disease remains controversial.

Although the available data is conflicting, there is recent evidence to support the use of BCAA supplementation in ESLD.[27,53–58] Some well-designed studies have shown that supplementation of diets with oral BCAA improved disease progression, hospital admission,[53] survival,[53,54] serum albumin concentration, and quality of life in cirrhotic patients[27,54] versus control subjects without supplementation. In a recent randomized pilot trial, early intervention with oral BCAA appeared to prolong the waiting period for liver transplantation by preserving hepatic reserve in cirrhosis.[55] All of these trials have lead to the consensus in recommending BCAA-enriched preparation for patients with chronic hepatic encephalopathy or intolerance to conventional proteins.[56–58] Recent ESPEN guidelines recommend that in patients with encephalopathy III or IV, the use of products enriched in BCAAs and low in AAA should be considered.[40]

Micronutrients

Nutritional therapy in patients with ESLD should not only focus on treatment of protein-calorie malnutrition, but should also aim to identify and correct micronutrient deficiencies. Micronutrient deficiencies are commonly seen in patients with advanced liver disease. For instance, patients with alcoholic cirrhosis who continue to consume alcohol are particularly at risk for developing water-soluble vitamin (ie, thiamine, folate) and magnesium deficiencies.[59] However, deficiencies in water-soluble vitamins also occur in nonalcoholic liver disease,[13] especially thiamine deficiency.[60]

Besides water-soluble vitamin deficiencies, fat-soluble vitamin (A, D, E, and K) deficiencies are also common in patients with chronic liver failure, but particularly those with cholestasis.[61] Fat-soluble vitamin deficiencies result from fat malabsorption, as well as defective fat-soluble vitamins mobilization from the liver. Vitamin A (retinol) deficiency has been described in cirrhosis and is considered as a risk factor for development of cancer, including hepatocellular carcinoma.[62] Vitamin A deficiency can cause night blindness, which has been shown to improve with a dose up to 50,000 units per day of vitamin A supplementation for 4 to 12 weeks.[19,63] However, night blindness not responsive to vitamin A might result from concomitant zinc deficiency.[64]

Zinc deficiency has also been associated with chronic liver disease. The liver plays an important role in zinc homeostasis by serving as a rapidly exchanging repository for zinc storage.[65] Zinc deficiency commonly occurs in patients with cirrhosis and is considered to precipitate hepatic encephalopathy.[66–69] However, trials of zinc supplementation have shown inconsistent results.[70,71] Despite these mixed results, zinc supplementation is recommended for patients with hepatic encephalopathy that does not respond to standard treatment.[72] Zinc deficiency may alter taste sensation in some individuals, and administration of zinc may indirectly improve food intake and nutritional state.[19]

Vitamin D deficiency is also highly associated with chronic liver disease, resulting from malabsorption, reduced exposure to UV light (decreased outdoors skin exposure to sunlight), and insufficient dietary vitamin D. Researchers at the University of Tennessee in Memphis found approximately 92% of 118 chronic liver disease patients had vitamin D deficiency and at least one-third had severe vitamin D deficiency, especially common in cirrhotic patients.[73] Vitamin D deficiency leads to decreased intestinal calcium and phosphorus absorption, eventually osteomalacia or osteoporosis as a result of calcium deficiency. Therefore, correction of vitamin D insufficiency with vitamin D_3 (800 IU/d) and calcium (1 gm/d) is recommended in all patients with chronic liver disease, especially in those at risk for osteoporosis.[74] However, higher doses may be warranted to normalize blood 25-hydroxyvitamin D levels, which should be monitored serially.

SUMMARY

The intention of this article is to increase the clinician's awareness of the unique metabolic abnormalities, as well as the effect and incidence of malnutrition accompanying ESLD. Protein-calorie malnutrition is an important complication of advanced liver disease with prognostic implications. Early and ongoing nutritional interventions can help to delay clinical deterioration, reduce the risk of complications, and improve survival. Careful nutrition and metabolic assessment can help evaluate and ensure optimal nutrition support goals. Nutritional therapy should focus on maintaining adequate protein and caloric intake and correcting micronutrient deficiencies.

REFERENCES

1. Merli M, Riggio O, Capocaccia L. Nutritional status in cirrhosis. J Hepatol 1994; 21:317–25.
2. Caregaro L, Alberino F, Amodio P, et al. Malnutrition in alcoholic and virus-related cirrhosis. Am J Clin Nutr 1996;63:602–9.
3. Campillo B, Richardet JP, Scherman E, et al. Evaluation of nutritional practice in hospitalized cirrhotic patients: results of a prospective study. Nutrition 2003;19: 515–21.
4. McCullough AJ, Bugianesi E. Protein-calorie malnutrition and the etiology of cirrhosis. Am J Gastroenterol 1997;92:734–8.
5. Thukuvath PJ, Triger DR. Evaluation of nutritional status by using anthropometry in adults with alcoholic and non-alcoholic liver disease. Am J Clin Nutr 1994;602: 269–73.
6. Alberino F, Gatta A, Amodio P, et al. Nutrition and survival in patients with liver cirrhosis. Nutrition 2001;17:445–50.
7. Kalman DR, Saltzman JR. Nutrition status predicts survival in cirrhosis. Nutr Rev 1996;54:217–9.
8. Selberg O, Bottcher J, Tusch G, et al. Identification of high- and low-risk patients before liver transplantation: a prospective cohort study of nutritional and metabolic parameters in 150 patients. Hepatology 1997;25:652–7.
9. Merli M, Riggio O, Dally L, et al. Does malnutrition affect survival in cirrhosis? PINC (Policentrica Italiana Nutrizione Cirrosi). Hepatology 1996;23:1041–6.
10. Prijatmoko D, Strauss BJ, Lambert JR, et al. Early detection of protein depletion in alcoholic cirrhosis: role of body composition analysis. Gastroenterology 1993; 105:1839–54.
11. Plauth M, Merli M, Kondrup J, et al. ESPEN guidelines for nutrition in liver disease and transplantation. Clin Nutr 1997;16:43–55.
12. DiCecco SR, Wieners EJ, Wiesner RH, et al. Assessment of nutritional status of patients with end-stage liver disease undergoing liver transplantation. Mayo Clin Proc 1989;64:95–102.
13. Cabre A, Gassull MA. Nutritional aspects of chronic liver disease. Clin Nutr 1993; 12:s52–63.
14. McClain CJ, Marsano L, Burk RF, et al. Trace metals in liver disease. Semin Liver Dis 1991;11:321–39.
15. Somi MH, Rahimi AO, Moshrefi B, et al. Nutritional status and blood trace elements in cirrhotic patients. Hepatitis Monthly 2007;7:27–32.

16. Zaina FE, Parolin MB, Lopes RW, et al. Prevalence of malnutrition in liver transplant candidates. Transplant Proc 2004;36:923–5.
17. Ferancheck AP, Gralla J, Ramirez RO, et al. Comparison of indices of vitamin A status in children with chronic liver disease. Hepatology 2005;42:782–92.
18. Delich PC, Siepler JK, Parker P. Liver disease. In: Gottschlich MM, DeLegge MH, Mattox T, et al, editors. The ASPEN nutrition support core curriculum: a case-based approach—the adult patient. Maryland: American Society of Parenteral and Enteral Nutrition (ASPEN); 2007. p. 547–57.
19. Garrett-Laser M, Russell RM, Jacques PF. Impairment of taste and olfaction in patients with cirrhosis: the role of vitamin A. Hum Nutr Clin Nutr 1984;38: 203–14.
20. Plauth M, Schutz ET. Cachexia in liver cirrhosis. Int J Cardiol 2002;85:83–7.
21. Testa R, Franceschini R, Giannini E, et al. Serum leptin levels in patients with viral chronic hepatitis or liver cirrhosis. J Hepatol 2000;33:33–7.
22. Gunnarsdottir SA, Sadik R, Shev S, et al. Small intestinal motility disturbances and bacterial overgrowth in patients with liver cirrhosis and portal hypertension. Am J Gastroenterol 2003;98:1362–70.
23. Conn HO. Is protein-losing enteropathy a significant complication of portal hypertension. Am J Gastroenterol 1998;93:127–8.
24. Muller NJ, Lautz HU, Plogmann B, et al. Energy expenditure and substrate oxidation in patients with cirrhosis: the impact of cause, clinical staging and nutritional state. Hepatology 1992;15:782–94.
25. Chang WK, Chao YC, Tang HS, et al. Effect of extra-carbohydrate supplementation in the late evening on energy expenditure and substrate oxidation in patients with liver cirrhosis. JPEN J Parenter Enteral Nutr 1997;21:96–9.
26. McCllough AJ, Tavill AS. Disordered energy and protein metabolism in liver disease. Semin Liver Dis 1991;11:265–77.
27. Khanna S, Gopalan S. Role of branched-chain amino acids in liver disease: the evidence for and against. Curr Opin Clin Nutr Metab Care 2007;10:297–303.
28. Peng S, Plank LD, McCall JL, et al. Body composition, muscle function, and energy expenditure in patients with liver cirrhosis: a comprehensive study. Am J Clin Nutr 2007;85:1257–66.
29. Muller MJ, Bottcher J, Selberg O, et al. Hypermetabolism in clinically stable patients with liver cirrhosis. Am J Clin Nutr 1999;69:1194–201.
30. Kondrup J. Nutrition in end stage liver disease. Best Pract Res Clin Gastroenterol 2006;20:547–60.
31. Scolapio JS, Bowen J, Stoner G, et al. Substrate oxidation in patients with cirrhosis: comparison with other nutritional markers. JPEN J Parenter Enteral Nutr 2000;24:150–3.
32. Kondrup J, Allison SP, Elia M, et al. ESPEN guidelines for nutrition screening 2002. Clin Nutr 2003;22:415–21.
33. Cabre E, Gassull MA. Nutrition in chronic liver disease and liver transplantation. Curr Opin Clin Nutr Metab Care 1998;1:423–30.
34. Russell MK, Mueller C. Nutrition screening and assessment. In: Gottschlich MM, DeLegge MH, Mattox T, et al, editors. The ASPEN nutrition support core curriculum: a case-based approach—the adult patient. Maryland: American Society of Parenteral and Enteral Nutrition (ASPEN); 2007. p. 163–86.
35. Alvares-da-Silva MR, Reverbel da Silveira T. Comparison between handgrip strength, subjective global assessment and prognostic nutritional index in assessing malnutrition and predicting outcome in cirrhotic outpatients. Nutrition 2005;21:113–7.

36. Schloerb PR, Forster J, Delcore R, et al. Bioelectrical impedance in the clinical evaluation of liver disease. Am J Clin Nutr 1996;64:S510–4.
37. Zillikens MC, van den Berg JW, Wilson JH, et al. The validity of bioelectrical impedance analysis in estimating total body water in patients with cirrhosis. J Hepatol 1992;16:59–65.
38. Morgan MY, Madden AM, Soulsby GT, et al. Derivation and validation of a new global method for assessing nutritional status in patients with cirrhosis. Hepatology 2006;44:823–35.
39. Plauth M, Cabre E, Riggio O, et al. ESPEN guidelines on enteral nutrition: liver disease. Clin Nutr 2006;25:285–94.
40. Plauth M, Cabre E, Campillo B, et al. ESPEN guidelines on parenteral nutrition: hepatology. Clin Nutr 2009;28:436–44.
41. Cordoba J, Lopez-Hellin J, Planas M, et al. Normal protein diet for episodic hepatic encephalopathy results of a randomized study. J Hepatol 2004;41:38–43.
42. Riordan SM, Williams R. Treatment of hepatic encephalopathy. N Engl J Med 1997;337:473–9.
43. Kondrop J, Muller MJ. Energy and protein requirements of patients with chronic liver disease. J Hepatol 1997;27:239–47.
44. Miwa Y, Shirakia M, Katoa M, et al. Improvement of fuel metabolism by nocturnal energy supplementation in patients with liver cirrhosis. Hepatol Res 2000;18:184–9.
45. Nompleggi DJ, Bonkovsky HL. Nutritional supplementation in chronic liver disease: an analytical review. Hepatology 1994;74:557–67.
46. Cabre E, Gonzelz-Huix F, Abad A, et al. Effect of total enteral nutrition on the short-term outcome of severely malnourished cirrhotics: a randomized controlled trial. Gastroenterology 1990;98:715–20.
47. Kearns PJ, Young H, Barcia G, et al. Accelerated improvement of alcoholic liver disease with enteral nutrition. Gastroenterology 1992;102:200–5.
48. Hirsch S, Bunout D, De la Maza P, et al. Controlled trial on nutrition supplementation in outpatient with symptomatic alcoholic cirrhosis. JPEN J Parenter Enteral Nutr 1993;17:119–24.
49. Loser C, Aschl G, Hebuterne X, et al. ESPEN guidelines on artificial enteral nutrition-percutaneous endoscopic gastrostomy (PEG). Clin Nutr 2005;24: 848–61.
50. Wicks C, Somasundaram S, Bjarnason I, et al. Comparison of enteral feeding and total parenteral nutrition after liver transplantation. Lancet 1994;344:837–40.
51. Plauth M, Roske AE, Romaniuk P, et al. Post-feeing hyperammonaemia in patients with transjugular intrahepatic portosystemic shunt and liver cirrhosis: role of small intestinal ammonia release and route of nutrient administration. Gut 2000;46:849–55.
52. Grau T, Bonet A, Rubio M, et al. Liver dysfunction associated with artificial nutrition in critically ill patients. Crit Care 2007;11:R10.
53. Marchesini G, Bianchi G, Merli M, et al. Nutritional supplementation with branched-chain amino acids in advanced cirrhosis: a double-blind, randomized trial. Gastroenterology 2003;124:1792–801.
54. Charlton M. Branched-chain amino acid granules: can they improve survival in patients with liver cirrhosis? Nat Clin Pract Gastroenterol Hepatol 2006;3:72–3.
55. Kawamura E, Habu D, Morikawa H, et al. Links a randomized pilot trial of oral branched-chain amino acids in early cirrhosis: validation using prognostic markers for pre-liver transplant status. Liver Transpl 2009;15:790–7.
56. Marchesini G, Dioguardi FS, Bianci G, et al. Long-term oral branched-chain amino acid treatment in chronic hepatic encephalopathy: a randomized double-blind casein-controlled trial. J Hepatol 1990;11:92–101.

57. Als-Nielsen B, Koretz RL, Gluud LL, et al. Branched-chain amino acid for hepatic encephalopathy. Cochrane Database Syst Rev 2003;3:CD001939.

58. Olde Damink SW, Jalan R, Deutz NE, et al. Isoleucine infusion during "simulated" upper gastrointestinal bleeding improves liver and muscle protein synthesis in cirrhotic patients. Hepatology 2007;45:560–8.

59. Leevy CM, Moroianu SA. Nutritional aspects of alcoholic liver disease. Clin Liver Dis 2005;9:67–81.

60. Levy S, Herve C, Delacoux E, et al. Thiamine deficiency in hepatitis C virus and alcohol-related liver disease. Dig Dis Sci 2002;47:543–8.

61. Sokol RJ. Fat-soluble vitamins and their importance in patients with cholestatic liver disease. Gastroenterol Clin North Am 1994;23:673–705.

62. Newsome PN, Beldon I, Moussa Y, et al. Low serum retinol levels are associated with hepatocellular carcinoma in patients with chronic liver disease. Aliment Pharmacol Ther 2000;14:1295–301.

63. Janczeska I, Ericzon BG, Eriksson LS. Influence of orthotopic liver transplantation on serum vitamin A levels in patient with chronic liver disease. Scand J Gastroenterol 1995;30:68–71.

64. Lieber CS. Alcohol: its metabolism and interaction with nutrient. Annu Rev Nutr 2000;20:395–430.

65. Krebs NE, Hambidge KM. Zinc metabolism and homeostasis: the application of tracer techniques to human zinc physiology. Biometals 2001;14:397–412.

66. Grungreiff K, Grungreiff S, Reinhold D. Zinc deficiency and hepatic encephalopathy: results of a long-term follow-up on zinc supplementation. J Trace Elem Exp Med 2000;13:21–31.

67. Van der Rijt CC, Schalm SW, Schat H, et al. Overt hepatic encephalopathy precipitated by zinc deficiency. Gastroenterology 1991;100:1114–8.

68. Yang SS, Lai YC, Chiang TR, et al. Role of zinc in subclinical hepatic encephalopahty: comparison with somatosensory-evoked potentials. J Gastroenterol Hepatol 2004;19:375–9.

69. Romero-Gomez M, Boza F, Garcia-Valdecasas MS, et al. Subclinical hepatic encephalopathy predicts the development of overt hepatic encephalopathy. Am J Gastroenterol 2001;96:2718–23.

70. Riggio O, Ariosto F, Merli M, et al. Short-term oral zinc supplementation does not improve chronic hepatic encephalopathy. Results of a double-blind crossover trial. Dig Dis Sci 1991;36:1204–8.

71. Marchesini G, Bugianesi E, Ronchi M, et al. Zinc supplementation and amino acid-nitrogen metabolism in patients with advanced cirrhosis. Hepatology 2003;23:1084–92.

72. Blei AT, Cordoba J, Practice Parameters Committee of the American College of Gastroenterology. Hepatic encephalopahty. Am J Gastroenterol 2001;96:1968–76.

73. American College of Gastroenterology. Vitamin D deficiency common in patients with IBD, chronic liver disease. 73rd Annual Scientific Meeting of the American College of Gastroenterology, October 2008. Available at: http://www.gi.org/media/releases/2008am/ACG08VitaminDDeficiency.pdf. Accessed November 11, 2009.

74. Collier JD, Ninkovic M, Compston JE. Guidelines on the management of osteoporosis associated with liver disease. Gut 2002;50(Suppl 1):i1–9.

Medical Management of Variceal Hemorrhage

Tram B. Cat, PharmD, BCPS[a],*, Xi Liu-DeRyke, PharmD[b]

KEYWORDS

- Variceal bleeding • Vasoactive therapy
- Upper gastrointestinal bleeding • Octreotide • Vasopressin
- Medical management

Gastroesophageal variceal hemorrhage is a major complication of portal hypertension in 50% to 60% of patients with liver cirrhosis and is a frequent cause of mortality in these patients.[1–3] The prevalence of variceal hemorrhage is approximately 5% to 15% yearly, and early variceal rebleeding has a rate of occurrence of 30% to 40% within the first 6 weeks.[4,5] The 1-year survival rate of patients after variceal hemorrhage was previously reported to be approximately 32% to 80%.[6,7] With the advent of new and improved therapeutic modalities over the past 2 decades, however, the age-adjusted in-hospital mortality rate has decreased by 45.4%.[1] Overall, the mortality rate associated with each episode of acute variceal hemorrhage has decreased to approximately 20%.[8] Unfortunately, more than 50% of patients who survive after the first bleeding episode will experience recurrent bleeding within 1 year.

Management of gastroesophageal varices should include prevention of initial and recurrent bleeding episodes and control of active hemorrhage. Therapies used in the management of gastroesophageal variceal hemorrhage may include pharmacologic therapy (vasoactive agents, nonselective β-blockers, and antibiotic prophylaxis), endoscopic therapy, transjugular intrahepatic portosystemic shunt (TIPS), and shunt surgery. This article focuses primarily on pharmacologic management of acute variceal hemorrhage.

RISK FACTORS AND PROGNOSIS

Varices are present in approximately 50% of patients diagnosed with liver cirrhosis.[5] Varices are characterized as portosystemic collaterals that result from dilated preexisting vascular channels caused by portal hypertension. Varices form when the hepatic

Financial disclosure: The authors have no financial interest to disclose.
[a] Critical Care, Department of Pharmacy, Antelope Valley Hospital, 1600 West Avenue, Lancaster, CA 93534, USA
[b] Department of Pharmacy, Orlando Regional Medical Center, 1414 Kuhl Avenue, MP 180, Orlando, FL 32806, USA
* Corresponding author.
E-mail address: tram.cat@avhospital.org

Crit Care Nurs Clin N Am 22 (2010) 381–393
doi:10.1016/j.ccell.2010.02.004
0899-5885/10/$ – see front matter © 2010 Elsevier Inc. All rights reserved.
ccnursing.theclinics.com

venous pressure gradient (HVPG) is 12 mm Hg or greater.[9,10] HVPG is the difference between the wedged hepatic vein pressures (WHVP) and free hepatic venous pressure (FHVP). When the HVPG is reduced to more than 20% from baseline, the risk for bleeding decreases significantly.[11]

Several risk factors have been associated with acute variceal hemorrhage mortality: low hematocrit level, high aminotransferase levels, HVPG greater than 12 mm Hg, presence of portal vein thrombosis, alcoholic liver disease, elevated serum bilirubin, low albumin levels, hepatic encephalopathy, hepatocellular carcinoma (HCC), and the Child-Turcotte-Pugh (CTP) score.[8] Additionally, an esophagogastroduodenoscopy screen is recommended when cirrhosis is diagnosed because active bleeding at initial endoscopy has been identified as a risk factor associated with mortality in these patients.

Traditionally, the CTP score has been used to stratify patients at risk for death after acute variceal hemorrhage, with a higher CTP score associated with an increased mortality. However, limitations of the CTP classification system include subjective parameters, such as ascites and encephalopathy, and the lack of standardization measurements of albumin and prothrombin time.

Since the model for end-stage liver disease (MELD) score was introduced, its accuracy in predicting 3-month mortality in patients with chronic liver disease after undergoing TIPS has been shown to be superior to the CTP classification system. In a randomized prospective trial of 256 patients with acute variceal hemorrhage, patients with MELD score of 18 or greater were at increased risk for dying within 6 weeks, and for rebleeding within the first 5 days after acute variceal hemorrhage ($P<.001$ and $P = .04$, respectively). Furthermore, patients with MELD score of 18 or greater either requiring 4 or more units of packed red blood cells (PRBC) within the first 24 hours of acute variceal hemorrhage (hazard ratio [HR], 11.3; $P<.001$) or who had active bleeding at endoscopy (HR, 9.9, $P<.001$) were at increased risk for death within 6 weeks of acute variceal hemorrhage.[8]

Independent predictors of mortality for acute variceal hemorrhage include increased prothrombin time, coexisting digestive carcinoma, use of corticosteroid, occurrence of upper gastrointestinal hemorrhage in an inpatient, hematemesis, and age older than 60 years.[12] Predictors of variceal hemorrhage include physical (elastic properties of the vessel, intravariceal/intraluminal pressure, variceal wall tension), clinical (continued alcohol use, severity of liver disease classified by Child-Pugh class A–C, presence of ascites), endoscopic (large varices, red wale markings), and hemodynamic factors (HVPG >12 mm Hg).[5] The most important predictor of hemorrhage is the size of varices (>5 mm). Similarly, rebleeding after acute variceal hemorrhage usually depends on the severity of the bleed and characteristics of the ulcer. Lee and colleagues[4] discovered that the incidence of infection and number of esophageal variceal ligations were significantly associated with higher rebleeding rates. Additionally, the rebleeding group was associated with higher mortality rates. Therefore, prevention of rebleeding could play a major role in reducing the rate of mortality in patients with cirrhosis and acute variceal hemorrhage.

PREVENTIVE THERAPY
Primary Prevention

Prophylactic therapy is a vital part of esophageal variceal management because bleeding (both first and recurrent episodes) is associated with high morbidity and mortality. If patients have a large varices, red wale marks at the base, or cirrhosis with Child-Pugh class B or C, primary prophylactic therapy is recommended.[13–15]

Both pharmacologic and nonpharmacologic therapies have been studied for primary prevention. Nonselective β-blockers (eg, propranolol, nadolol) are the first-line pharmacologic therapy for primary prevention of variceal hemorrhage. Nonselective β-blockers can reduce the HVPG through β-1 blockade, and also reduce splanchnic collateral flow through β-2 vasoconstriction. A meta-analysis reported that, compared with placebo, nonselective β-blockers were associated with an absolute risk reduction (ARR) of 10% in preventing the first variceal bleeding.[16] A reduction in 2-year mortality was also shown (ARR, 4%), although not statistically significant. The goal of using a nonselective β-blocker is to achieve a 25% reduction of heart rate from baseline, or less than 55 beats per minute.[13,14]

Other pharmacologic agents that have been studied for prophylactic therapy include nitrates and spironolactone. Isosorbide mononitrate (ISMN) is a potent veno- and arterial vasodilator, which can reduce portal pressure. However, its use was associated with no difference in the incidence of primary bleeding, but a higher mortality (72%) was seen in the ISMN group in patients older than 50 years compared with the propranolol group (48%; $P = .006$).[17] Similar findings were reported in a double-blind, randomized clinical trial of 349 patients with an endoscopic-confirmed variceal of any size. Significantly more patients experienced adverse events (primarily headache) in the group treated with ISMN plus propranolol compared with the propranolol-alone group.

Spironolactone is an antialdosterone diuretic that can reduce plasma volume and splanchnic blood flow, therefore lowering portal pressure. A preliminary study evaluated the efficacy of combining nadolol with spironolactone in the primary prevention of variceal hemorrhage.[18] Again, combination therapy was no more efficacious than nadolol alone. Based on these results, ISMN and spironolactone are not recommended for primary prevention because of higher side effects and no advantages associated with their efficacy.

Endoscopic band ligation (EBL) is a nonpharmacologic option for the primary prevention of variceal hemorrhage. Several meta-analyses have been conducted to evaluate whether pharmacologic intervention or EBL is better in preventing bleeding and mortality.[19,20] Khuroo and colleagues[20] showed a significant reduction in the incidence of primary hemorrhage in patients treated with EBL compared with those treated with β-blockers ($P = .034$), with a mean follow-up of 12 to 22 months. No difference in mortality was observed between the groups. Another recent meta-analysis, however, failed to find a difference in either the incidence of primary hemorrhage or mortality, with a median follow-up of 20 months.[19] In the regression analysis, the authors found that duration of follow-up was a significant predictor of treatment success (the shorter the follow-up, the more effective the treatment seemed), which may explain the significant findings from the previous meta-analysis by Khuroo and colleagues.[20] When the cost-effectiveness of EBL and β-blocker therapy was examined, EBL was more cost-effective when the quality of life was considered but not when cost per life year was considered.[21] Therefore, current guidelines recommend both therapies as first-line therapy for primary prevention.[13]

The advantages of β-blocker therapy are the low cost and tolerability of the medications. Additionally, β-blocker therapy has been shown to decrease the incidence of spontaneous bacterial peritonitis.[22] Because β-blockers are a lifelong therapy, compliance is often a problem because of side effects such as dyspnea, bronchospasm, fatigue, and decreased sexual activity. EBL provides a better compliance rate and few systemic side effects. However, EBL does not prevent gastric bleeding, and procedure-related bleeding can occur. Unlike β-blocker therapy, patients receiving EBL require frequent esophagogastroduodenoscopy follow-ups.[13]

Secondary Prevention

Because the recurrence rate of hemorrhage in patients who survive their first variceal hemorrhage is as high as 50%, secondary prophylaxis against rebleeding is essential in the management of acute variceal hemorrhage. Even though either β-blockers or EBL alone is effective in preventing rebleeding, studies have shown that the combination of β-blockers and EBL is superior to either therapy alone.[23–25] In a prospective randomized trial, EBL alone was compared with combination therapy consisting of EBL with nadolol and sucralfate for managing rebleeding in 122 patients with a history of variceal bleeding. Results showed a significant reduction in the incidence of rebleeding in the combination group compared with the EBL-alone group (23% vs 47%, respectively; $P<.01$).[25]

Another multicentered randomized trial comparing EBL alone versus EBL plus nadolol immediately after acute variceal hemorrhage for secondary prophylaxis showed a rebleeding rate of 14% in the combination group compared with 38% in the EBL-alone group ($P = .006$).[23] However, more patients experienced adverse effects in the combination group. A recent meta-analysis of 23 randomized controlled trials assessing the efficacy of combined endoscopic therapy with medical management for secondary prophylaxis showed that combination therapy was more effective than either endoscopic therapy or drug therapy alone in preventing rebleeding.[24] Therefore, EBL plus nonselective β-blockers are the first-line option in the secondary prevention after acute variceal hemorrhage.[13] Shunt surgery or TIPS should be considered in patients for whom combination therapy fails.

MEDICAL TREATMENT

Although endoscopic or surgical intervention (TIPS or shunt surgery) is warranted for controlling active bleeding, pharmacologic therapy (vasoactive agents) should be initiated promptly and continued for several days after definitive treatment because of the high incidence of recurrent bleeding and mortality after initial hemorrhage. **Fig. 1** outlines a suggested algorithm for the management of acute variceal hemorrhage. Several vasoactive agents, including vasopressin, terlipressin, somatostatin, and octreotide, have been studied in the management of acute variceal hemorrhage. Only vasopressin and octreotide are available in the United States.

Vasopressin

Vasopressin decreases portal blood flow and pressure through splanchnic vasoconstriction and has been used for the management of upper gastrointestinal bleeding since the 1960s. Early experience with vasopressin was mixed regarding the efficacy in controlling active bleeding, whereas significant systemic complications such as myocardial ischemia/infarction and bowel ischemia have been reported (**Table 1**).[26–29] Subsequently, the vasodilator nitroglycerin has been shown to help minimize these systemic complications. Two randomized trials showed that the addition of nitroglycerin significantly reduced systemic complications with vasopressin therapy; however, no benefit was shown in rebleeding rate and mortality.[27,28] Because of the availability of octreotide and the known serious adverse effects and lack of clear benefit associated with vasopressin, combination therapy with vasopressin and nitroglycerin is no longer the mainstay of vasoactive treatment.

Octreotide

Octreotide, a synthetic somatostatin analog, has become a preferred agent for adjunctive therapy in the immediate control of variceal bleeding because of its safety

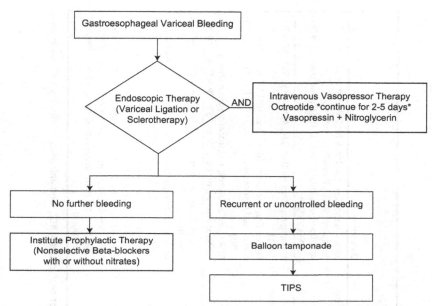

Fig. 1. Suggested algorithm for management of acute variceal hemorrhage. TIPS, transjugular intrahepatic portosystemic shunt.

and efficacy profile compared with alternative therapies (**Table 2**).[30–41] Octreotide decreases portal blood flow and pressures through both direct splanchnic vasoconstriction and splanchnic vasodilation by inhibiting glucagon release.

When compared with placebo, octreotide infusion (median treatment, 120 h) was more effective in controlling bleed ($P = .02$).[16] In a meta-analysis of trials evaluating the safety and efficacy of octreotide for esophageal variceal hemorrhage, it was comparable to sclerotherapy in controlling bleed (relative risk [RR], 0.94; 95% CI, 0.55–1.62) but showed favorable outcomes in sustained control of bleeding compared with vasopressin or terlipressin (RR, 0.58; 95% CI, 0.42–0.81).[42] Furthermore, octreotide showed a borderline mortality benefit compared with any alternative therapy (vasopressin/terlipressin, placebo/no therapy, and sclerotherapy; RR, 0.76; 95% CI, 0.58–1.0; test for homogeneity, $P = .86$).[42]

In another meta-analysis, Gross and colleagues[43] also showed that initial control of bleeding was similar between sclerotherapy and vasoactive therapy (octreotide or somatostatin), with vasoactive therapy slightly more efficient at controlling bleed than vasoconstrictive therapy (vasopressin or terlipressin). Ligation therapy, however, was significantly more successful in controlling bleed than vasoactive therapy ($P<.02$). The complications associated with either sclerotherapy or ligation are small.[2] However, sclerotherapy can cause important local complications, such as perforation, ulceration, and stricture. Ligation therapy causes even fewer complications, which may include superficial ulcerations and rare formations of strictures.

Octreotide has been shown to have fewer major complications than vasopressin (RR, 0.31; 95% CI, 0.11–0.87) and had a similar complication profile to no intervention/placebo (RR, 1.06; 95% CI, 0.72–1.55).[42] Major complications were described as arrhythmias, hyper/hypotension, cardiac or intestinal ischemia, pneumonia, pulmonary edema, or any adverse effect requiring termination of treatment.

Table 1
Vasopressin therapy for variceal hemorrhage

Study	Design	Interventions	Outcomes
Fogel et al[26]	RCT VP: 14 patients P: 19 patients	VP: 40 U/h until bleeding controlled, then 20 U/h Total infusion × 24 h	Initial hemostasis (within 6 h): 29% VP vs 32% P Mortality: 50% VP vs 42% P (NS) ADR (cardiovascular changes; abdominal cramps): 41% VP vs 29% P
Tsai et al[27]	RCT VP: 19 patients VP-NTG: 20 patients	VP: 0.66 U/min, then 0.33 U/min × 24 h Identical VP dosing with NTG, 0.6 mg, sublingual every 30 min for first 6 h	Initial hemostasis (within 6 h): 47% VP vs 55% VP-NTG (NS) Rebleeding occurred: 26% VP vs 10% VP-NTG (NS) Completed hemostasis in 24 h: 21% VP vs 45% VP-NTG (NS) ADR (cardiac events; electrocardiogram changes; abdominal pain): 89% VP vs 35% VP-NTG (P<.001)
Gimson et al[28]	RCT VP: 30 patients VP-NTG: 32 patients	VP: 20 U bolus, then 0.4 U/min × 12 h Identical VP dosing with NGT 40 μg/min × 12 h	Control of bleeding at 12 h: 44% VP vs 68% VP-NTG (P<.05) Withdraw therapy because of ADR (cardiac events): 23% VP vs 3% VP-NTG (P<.02)
Huang et al[29]	P, RCT Oct: 20 patients VP: 21 patients	Oct: 100 μg bolus, then 25 μg/h VP: 0.4 U/min over 24 h	Initial hemostasis (within 6 h): 75% Oct vs 62% VP (NS) Rebleeding occurred: 15% Oct vs 29% VP (NS) Complete hemostasis in 24 h: 60% Oct vs 33% VP (NS) ADR: 15% Oct (abdominal fullness or nausea); 38% VP (abdominal pain, bradycardia, chest pain, ischemic purpura)

Abbreviations: ADR, adverse drug reactions; NS, not significant; NTG, nitroglycerin; Oct, octreotide; P, placebo; RCT, randomized controlled trial; VP, vasopressin; VP-NTG, vasopressin plus nitroglycerin.

Although these major adverse effects are concerns with octreotide use, hyperglycemia is the most common adverse effects. Other side effects associated with octreotide are headache, diarrhea, abdominal discomfort, nausea, and injection site pain. These complications, however, are generally not seen with 3 to 5 days of therapy.

Octreotide combined with endoscopic therapy is the preferred first-line treatment for producing hemostasis. Besson and colleagues[37] showed that the combination of octreotide and sclerotherapy had a greater patient survival rate without rebleeding than sclerotherapy alone for active variceal bleeding (87% vs 71%; $P = .009$). Other studies have also obtained favorable outcomes in decreased rebleeding rates when octreotide was combined with endoscopic therapy.[38,40]

When using octreotide for acute variceal bleeding, the most commonly recommended administration schedule is an initial 50-μg intravenous bolus followed by a continuous intravenous infusion at 50 μg/h for 5 days. Single therapy with octreotide in the management of variceal bleeding is controversial because of the rapid development of tachyphylaxis. In a dose-finding study investigating the hemodynamic effects of intravenous octreotide administration, Escorsell and colleagues[44] reported that continuous octreotide infusion resulted in rapid development of desensitization or tachyphylaxis phenomenon. Similar results were observed when octreotide was administered as repeated boluses, with additional boluses eliciting half the effects of the previous bolus dose on HVPG. These results may explain differences in outcomes associated with octreotide.

Proton Pump Inhibitors

Many theories support the use of proton pump inhibitors (PPIs) in patients with cirrhosis to prevent against peptic complications secondary to variceal or hypertensive gastropathic bleeding.[45] First, an increased prevalence of peptic ulcers in patients with cirrhosis may be a consequence of portal hypertension. In the presence of ascites and water retention found in these patients, acid reflux could be exacerbated and may contribute to esophagitis and variceal bleeding. In addition, some studies showed that patients with cirrhosis and *Helicobacter pylori* infection had an increased risk for developing ulcers. However, conflicting studies show that eradication of *H pylori* does not seem to prevent gastroduodenal ulcer formation and bleeding in patients with cirrhosis. Lastly, endoscopic treatment for variceal bleeding or prevention of bleeding varices may produce esophageal motility dysfunction and result in acid-related reflux esophagitis.

Unfortunately, scarce evidence shows the protective role of PPIs in the prevention and treatment of esophageal complications after endoscopic therapy of esophageal varices. One retrospective study evaluated the combination of pantoprazole and octreotide infusion for variceal bleeding.[46] Compared with octreotide infusion alone versus octreotide with short-term (<24 h) infusion of pantoprazole, or octreotide with intermittent acid suppression, combination therapy did not reduce the requirement of packed red blood cell–transfused endoscopic interventions or incidence of rebleeding. Furthermore, because the incidence of gastric variceal bleeding is small, routine use of PPIs is not currently recommended for managing active bleeding of esophageal varices.

FUTURE THERAPIES

Several other pharmacologic agents have been investigated for preventing and managing variceal hemorrhage. Carvedilol, a nonselective β-blocker with alpha-1

Table 2
Octreotide therapy for variceal hemorrhage

Study	Design	Medications	Outcomes
Octreotide vs vasopressin or terlipressin + nitroglycerin			
Hwang et al[30]	O, R N = 48	Oct, 100 µg × 1 then 25 µg/h; VP, 0.4 U/min (both × 24 h)	Initial bleeding control in first 6 h: 88% Oct vs 54% VP (P = .03); Bleeding control at 24 h: 63% Oct vs 46% VP (NS)
Silvain et al[31]	O, R N = 100	Oct, 25 µg/h × 12 h, then 100 µg SQ at 12 h and 18 h; TP, 2 mg IV × 1, then 1 mg q4h + transdermal NTG 10 mg × 12 h (both × 24 h)	Bleeding control at 12 h: 78% Oct vs 59% TP (NS); Fewer transfusions at 12 h in Oct group (P = .012)
Octreotide vs sclerotherapy or octreotide as adjunctive therapy			
Sung et al[32]	O, R N = 100	Oct, 50 µg × 1, then 50 µg/h × 48 h, then sclerotherapy; Sclerotherapy on admission	Bleeding control, episodes of rebleeding, transfusion between the groups (NS); Hospital length of stay and overall hospital mortality between the groups (NS)
Jenkins et al[33]	O, R N = 150	Oct, 50 µg/h × 48 h, then sclerotherapy; Emergency sclerotherapy	Control of bleeding between the groups (NS)
Sivri et al[34]	O, R N = 66	Oct, 50 µg × 1, then 50 µg/h × 12 h; Sclerotherapy	Bleeding control or rebleeding rate between the groups (NS); Transfusions and mortality between the groups (NS)
D'Amico et al[35]	DB, P, RCT N = 262	Oct, 100 µg SC 3x/d × 15 d with or without β-blockers and/or sclerotherapy	Reduction in rebleeding in patients receiving Oct with β-blockers and/or sclerotherapy (P = .03)
Freitas et al[36]	O, R N = 197	Group 1: Oct, 25 µg/h × 48 h or emergency sclerotherapy in patients with recent bleeding; Group 2: Oct, 25 µg/h × 48 h and/or emergency sclerotherapy in patients with active bleeding	Group 1: Bleeding control, transfusions, or mortality between therapies (NS); Group 2: Oct + sclerotherapy improved initial hemostasis (P<.001), hemostasis at 48 h (P<.04), transfusion requirements (P<.01)

Besson et al[37]	DB, P, RCT N = 199	Oct, 25 μg/h × 5 d P (after initial sclerotherapy)	Fewer patients without rebleeding in Oct group after 5 d ($P = .009$) Fewer transfusions at 24 h in Oct group ($P = .006$)
Sung et al[38]	O, R N = 94	Oct, 50 μg IV × 1, then 50 μg/h × 5 d + EBL EBL alone	Rebleeding rate: 9% Oct + EBL vs 38% EBL alone ($P<.0007$) Number of patients requiring tamponade for bleeding control: 1 patient in Oct + EBL vs 10 patients in EBL alone ($P = .0039$)
Primignani et al[39]	DB, P, RCT N = 58	Oct, 100 μg SC 3x/d × 29 d + sclerotherapy Sclerotherapy alone	Rebleeding rate or mortality between the groups (NS)
Zuberi and Baloch[40]	DB, P, RCT N = 70	Oct, 50 μg/h × 5 d P (after initial sclerotherapy)	A significant reduction in rebleeding rates ($P = 0.04$) or need for transfusions ($P = 0.03$) in Oct group
Morales et al[41]	P, PRCT N = 68	Group 1: Oct, 50 μg IV × 1, then 50 μg/h × 24 h, then 25 μg/h × 24 h Group 2: P (all patients initially underwent emergent sclerotherapy)	7-day mortality: 20% Oct vs 17.85% P (NS) Rebleeding rate: 20% Oct vs 21.4% P (NS) Mean number of blood transfusion units: 2.05 Oct vs 2.08 P (NS) Number of patients requiring intensive care unit stay: 20 of 40 Oct vs 10 of 28 P (NS)

Abbreviations: DB, double-blind; EBL, endoscopic band ligation; IV, intravenous; NS, not significant; NTG, nitroglycerin; O, open label; Oct, octreotide; P, placebo; PRCT, prospective randomized control trial; R, randomized; RCT, randomized control trial; SQ, subcutaneous; TP, terlipressin; VP, vasopressin.

blockade property may provide greater portal pressure reduction compared with other nonselective β-blockers.[47] In an intent-to-treat analysis, Tripathi and colleagues[48] prospectively evaluated carvedilol for primary prophylaxis compared with EBL in high-risk patients. They found that first variceal bleeding occurred in 10% of the carvedilol group compared with 23% of the EBL group ($P = .04$). No difference in mortality was noted between the groups. Although results from this preliminary study are promising, more data are needed before carvedilol can be recommended for primary or secondary prophylaxis.

Because liver cirrhosis is the most common cause of variceal bleeding, recombinant factor VIIa (rFVIIa; the most common deficient clotting factor) has been investigated as adjunctive therapy for the management of acute variceal hemorrhage.[49,50] Bosch and colleagues[50] randomized 237 patients into two groups receiving either eight doses of rFVIIa, 100 μg/kg, or placebo in addition to standard pharmacologic and endoscopic therapy. Overall, no significant differences were seen in control of bleeding within 24 hours, prevention of rebleeding, red blood cell transfusion, and mortality. Thromboembolic complications were also similar between the groups.

Similarly, a recent prospective, randomized trial of 256 patients evaluating the benefit and safety of rFVIIa in high-risk patients (Child-Pugh score >8) with acute variceal hemorrhage failed to show a difference between rFVIIa (300 or 600 μg/kg) and placebo in controlling bleed within 24 hours of acute variceal hemorrhage.[49] The rebleeding rate and mortality within 5 days of acute variceal hemorrhage were also no different. Therefore, routine use of rFVIIa for acute variceal hemorrhage management is not recommended.

SUMMARY

Patients with varices or acute variceal hemorrhage have high morbidity and mortality. Aggressive preventive management should be instituted after diagnosis. Although nonselective β-blockers are the first-line treatment for primary prevention of acute variceal hemorrhage, a combination of drug and endoscopic therapies is recommended for secondary prophylaxis against rebleeding. Prompt initiation of vasoactive therapy, such as octreotide, in conjunction with endoscopic or surgical intervention is the most rational approach in managing patients with active bleeding.

REFERENCES

1. Jamal MM, Samarasena JB, Hashemzadeh M. Decreasing in-hospital mortality for oesophageal variceal hemorrhage in the USA. Eur J Gastroenterol Hepatol 2008;20:947.
2. Sharara AI, Rockey DC. Gastroesophageal variceal hemorrhage. N Engl J Med 2001;345:669.
3. van Leerdam ME. Epidemiology of acute upper gastrointestinal bleeding. Best Pract Res Clin Gastroenterol 2008;22:209.
4. Lee SW, Lee TY, Chang CS. Independent factors associated with recurrent bleeding in cirrhotic patients with esophageal variceal hemorrhage. Dig Dis Sci 2009;54:1128.
5. Sass DA, Chopra KB. Portal hypertension and variceal hemorrhage. Med Clin North Am 2009;93:837.
6. Graham DY, Smith JL. The course of patients after variceal hemorrhage. Gastroenterology 1981;80:800.
7. Koransky JR, Galambos JT, Hersh T, et al. The mortality of bleeding esophageal varices in a private university hospital. Am J Surg 1978;136:339.

8. Bambha K, Kim WR, Pedersen R, et al. Predictors of early re-bleeding and mortality after acute variceal haemorrhage in patients with cirrhosis. Gut 2008;57:814.
9. Garcia-Tsao G, Groszmann RJ, Fisher RL, et al. Portal pressure, presence of gastroesophageal varices and variceal bleeding. Hepatology 1985;5:419.
10. Viallet A, Marleau D, Huet M, et al. Hemodynamic evaluation of patients with intra-hepatic portal hypertension. Relationship between bleeding varices and the por-tohepatic gradient. Gastroenterology 1975;69:1297.
11. Feu F, Garcia-Pagan JC, Bosch J, et al. Relation between portal pressure response to pharmacotherapy and risk of recurrent variceal haemorrhage in patients with cirrhosis. Lancet 1995;346:1056.
12. Chiu PW, Ng EK. Predicting poor outcome from acute upper gastrointestinal hemorrhage. Gastroenterol Clin North Am 2009;38:215.
13. Garcia-Tsao G, Lim JK. Management and treatment of patients with cirrhosis and portal hypertension: recommendations from the Department of Veterans Affairs Hepatitis C Resource Center Program and the National Hepatitis C Program. Am J Gastroenterol 2009;104:1802.
14. Garcia-Tsao G, Sanyal AJ, Grace ND, et al. Prevention and management of gastroesophageal varices and variceal hemorrhage in cirrhosis. Am J Gastroen-terol 2007;102:2086.
15. Villanueva C, Balanzo J. Variceal bleeding: pharmacological treatment and prophylactic strategies. Drugs 2008;68:2303.
16. D'Amico G, Pagliaro L, Bosch J. Pharmacological treatment of portal hyperten-sion: an evidence-based approach. Semin Liver Dis 1999;19:475.
17. Angelico M, Carli L, Piat C, et al. Effects of isosorbide-5-mononitrate compared with propranolol on first bleeding and long-term survival in cirrhosis. Gastroenter-ology 1997;113:1632.
18. Abecasis R, Kravetz D, Fassio E, et al. Nadolol plus spironolactone in the prophy-laxis of first variceal bleed in nonascitic cirrhotic patients: a preliminary study. Hepatology 2003;37:359.
19. Gluud LL, Klingenberg S, Nikolova D, et al. Banding ligation versus beta-blockers as primary prophylaxis in esophageal varices: systematic review of randomized trials. Am J Gastroenterol 2007;102:2842.
20. Khuroo MS, Khuroo NS, Farahat KL, et al. Meta-analysis: endoscopic variceal ligation for primary prophylaxis of oesophageal variceal bleeding. Aliment Phar-macol Ther 2005;21:347.
21. Imperiale TF, Klein RW, Chalasani N. Cost-effectiveness analysis of variceal ligation vs. beta-blockers for primary prevention of variceal bleeding. Hepatology 2007;45:870.
22. Turnes J, Garcia-Pagan JC, Abraldes JG, et al. Pharmacological reduction of portal pressure and long-term risk of first variceal bleeding in patients with cirrhosis. Am J Gastroenterol 2006;101:506.
23. de la Pena J, Brullet E, Sanchez-Hernandez E, et al. Variceal ligation plus nadolol compared with ligation for prophylaxis of variceal rebleeding: a multicenter trial. Hepatology 2005;41:572.
24. Gonzalez R, Zamora J, Gomez-Camarero J, et al. Meta-analysis: combination endoscopic and drug therapy to prevent variceal rebleeding in cirrhosis. Ann Intern Med 2008;149:109.
25. Lo GH, Lai KH, Cheng JS, et al. Endoscopic variceal ligation plus nadolol and sucralfate compared with ligation alone for the prevention of variceal rebleeding: a prospective, randomized trial. Hepatology 2000;32:461.
26. Fogel MR, Knauer CM, Andres LL, et al. Continuous intravenous vasopressin in active upper gastrointestinal bleeding. Ann Intern Med 1982;96:565.

27. Tsai YT, Lay CS, Lai KH, et al. Controlled trial of vasopressin plus nitroglycerin vs. vasopressin alone in the treatment of bleeding esophageal varices. Hepatology 1986;6:406.
28. Gimson AE, Westaby D, Hegarty J, et al. A randomized trial of vasopressin and vasopressin plus nitroglycerin in the control of acute variceal hemorrhage. Hepatology 1986;6:410.
29. Huang CC, Sheen IS, Chu CM, et al. A prospective randomized controlled trial of sandostatin and vasopressin in the management of acute bleeding esophageal varices. Changgeng Yi Xue Za Zhi 1992;15:78.
30. Hwang SJ, Lin HC, Chang CF, et al. A randomized controlled trial comparing octreotide and vasopressin in the control of acute esophageal variceal bleeding. J Hepatol 1992;16:320.
31. Silvain C, Carpentier S, Sautereau D, et al. Terlipressin plus transdermal nitroglycerin vs. octreotide in the control of acute bleeding from esophageal varices: a multicenter randomized trial. Hepatology 1993;18:61.
32. Sung JJ, Chung SC, Lai CW, et al. Octreotide infusion or emergency sclerotherapy for variceal haemorrhage. Lancet 1993;342:637.
33. Jenkins SA, Shields R, Davies M, et al. A multicentre randomised trial comparing octreotide and injection sclerotherapy in the management and outcome of acute variceal haemorrhage. Gut 1997;41:526.
34. Sivri B, Oksuzoglu G, Bayraktar Y, et al. A prospective randomized trial from Turkey comparing octreotide versus injection sclerotherapy in acute variceal bleeding. Hepatogastroenterology 2000;47:168.
35. D'Amico G, Politi F, Morabito A, et al. Octreotide compared with placebo in a treatment strategy for early rebleeding in cirrhosis. A double blind, randomized pragmatic trial. Hepatology 1998;28:1206.
36. Freitas DS, Sofia C, Pontes JM, et al. Octreotide in acute bleeding esophageal varices: a prospective randomized study. Hepatogastroenterology 2000;47:1310.
37. Besson I, Ingrand P, Person B, et al. Sclerotherapy with or without octreotide for acute variceal bleeding. N Engl J Med 1995;333:555.
38. Sung JJ, Chung SC, Yung MY, et al. Prospective randomised study of effect of octreotide on rebleeding from oesophageal varices after endoscopic ligation. Lancet 1995;346:1666.
39. Primignani M, Andreoni B, Carpinelli L, et al. Sclerotherapy plus octreotide versus sclerotherapy alone in the prevention of early rebleeding from esophageal varices: a randomized, double-blind, placebo-controlled, multicenter trial. New Italian Endoscopic Club. Hepatology 1995;21:1322.
40. Zuberi BF, Baloch Q. Comparison of endoscopic variceal sclerotherapy alone and in combination with octreotide in controlling acute variceal hemorrhage and early rebleeding in patients with low-risk cirrhosis. Am J Gastroenterol 2000;95:768.
41. Morales GF, Pereira Lima JC, Hornos AP, et al. Octreotide for esophageal variceal bleeding treated with endoscopic sclerotherapy: a randomized, placebo-controlled trial. Hepatogastroenterology 2007;54:195.
42. Corley DA, Cello JP, Adkisson W, et al. Octreotide for acute esophageal variceal bleeding: a meta-analysis. Gastroenterology 2001;120:946.
43. Gross M, Schiemann U, Muhlhofer A, et al. Meta-analysis: efficacy of therapeutic regimens in ongoing variceal bleeding. Endoscopy 2001;33:737.
44. Escorsell A, Bandi JC, Andreu V, et al. Desensitization to the effects of intravenous octreotide in cirrhotic patients with portal hypertension. Gastroenterology 2001;120:161.

45. Lodato F, Azzaroli F, Di Girolamo M, et al. Proton pump inhibitors in cirrhosis: tradition or evidence based practice? World J Gastroenterol 2008;14:2980.
46. Alaniz C, Mohammad RA, Welage LS. Continuous infusion of pantoprazole with octreotide does not improve management of variceal hemorrhage. Pharmacotherapy 2009;29:248.
47. Lin HC, Yang YY, Hou MC, et al. Acute administration of carvedilol is more effective than propranolol plus isosorbide-5-mononitrate in the reduction of portal pressure in patients with viral cirrhosis. Am J Gastroenterol 2004;99:1953.
48. Tripathi D, Ferguson JW, Kochar N, et al. Randomized controlled trial of carvedilol versus variceal band ligation for the prevention of the first variceal bleed. Hepatology 2009;50:825.
49. Bosch J, Thabut D, Albillos A, et al. Recombinant factor VIIa for variceal bleeding in patients with advanced cirrhosis: a randomized, controlled trial. Hepatology 2008;47:1604.
50. Bosch J, Thabut D, Bendtsen F, et al. Recombinant factor VIIa for upper gastrointestinal bleeding in patients with cirrhosis: a randomized, double-blind trial. Gastroenterology 2004;127:1123.

Acute Liver Failure

Tenita P. Foston, RN, MSN, FNP-C*, David Carpentar, MPAS, PA-C

KEYWORDS

- Acute liver failure • Multiple system failure
- Liver transplantation • Hepatitis

Acute liver failure (ALF) is an uncommon condition involving the rapid deterioration of liver functions and coagulation in previously well patients. The loss of liver function produces a cascade of systemic effects that rapidly overwhelm patients unless acted on. The key to managing patients with ALF revolves around having the resources and expertise to manage patients with rapidly evolving multiple system failure.

OVERVIEW

Although overall data are hard to extrapolate, ALF probably accounts for more than 2000 ICU admissions per year.[1] Before liver transplantation became commonly available, ALF had an extremely poor prognosis, with a survival rate of less than 15%. With the advent of liver transplantation in the past 15 years and improved intensive care management, survival rates are now in the 60% to 80% range.[2] Although important in the context of ALF, liver transplantation for ALF remains a small part of the overall transplant volume, at approximately 6%.[3,4]

ALF is generally defined as a coagulopathy disorders (international normalized ratio [INR] >1.5) and alteration of mental status (encephalopathy) in patients without known cirrhosis and in an illness of less than 26 weeks.[5] Certain diseases, such as Wilson disease, autoimmune hepatitis, and vertically acquired hepatitis B, may be included if their symptoms have been recognized for less than 26 weeks.[6] Several terms differentiating length of time between symptoms, such as jaundice and onset of encephalopathy, have been proposed. These terms generally divide the course into 3 periods: hyperacute, less than 7 days; acute, 7 to 21 days; and subacute, greater than 21 days and less than 26 weeks.

CAUSES

ALF can have various causes. Outcomes vary based on the cause.

Hepatic Viruses

The most common cause of acute viral hepatitis is hepatitis A, but this type of hepatitis rarely progresses to fulminant hepatic failure. Hepatitis B is more likely to cause

Emory University Hospital, 1364 Clifton Road NE, Atlanta, GA 30322, USA
* Corresponding author.
E-mail address: Tenita.Foston@emoryhealthcare.org

Crit Care Nurs Clin N Am 22 (2010) 395–402
doi:10.1016/j.ccell.2010.05.001
0899-5885/10/$ – see front matter © 2010 Elsevier Inc. All rights reserved.

a fulminant picture than the other viral hepatic diseases. It may even be classified as an acute-on-chronic disease process in patients who did not know they had hepatitis B and, for whatever reason, and began to have rapid liver decompensation. Hepatitis C, alternatively, rarely causes fulminant hepatic failure. Other viral causes of fulminant hepatic failure include hepatitis delta virus coinfection or superinfection, hepatitis E (especially in pregnant women in endemic areas), Epstein-Barr virus, cytomegalovirus, herpes simplex virus, and varicella zoster.[7]

Drug Toxicity

There are many drugs that may cause fulminant or subfulminant hepatic failure. The most common and most well known drug is acetaminophen by intentional or unintentional overdose. There is greater likelihood of hepatotoxicity from drugs in patients with depleted glutathione stores that occurs with chronic alcohol use. Fulminant hepatic failure due to acetaminophen toxicity generally has a relatively favorable outcome, and prognostic variables permit reasonable accuracy in determining the need for liver transplantation.[8] Patients who present with deep coma, greater than 6 arterial pH less than 7.3, significantly elevated creatinine (>3.4), or prolonged prothrombin time tend to have a poor prognosis.[8] Patients who present with less profound symptoms may have spontaneous recovery of the liver failure.

Prescription drugs can also cause fulminant or subfulminant hepatic failure. These drugs may include antibiotics, oral hypoglycemic agents, lipid-lowering medications, antidepressants, antiepileptics, and oral diabetic medications. Illicit drugs that may cause liver failure include ecstasy and cocaine. Herbal drugs that may also cause liver failure include ginseng, Teucrium polium, and kava-kava.

Metabolic

There are several metabolic disorders that may lead to ALF. Wilson disease is a process where there are elevated copper levels in the system. This disease is cured with liver transplantation. Acute fatty liver of pregnancy may resolve after delivery of a baby but may progress to need for liver transplantation. α_1-Antitrypsin deficiency, Reye syndrome, galactosemia, and fructose intolerance are also metabolic diseases that may cause ALF.

Autoimmue

Autoimmune hepatitis is another disease process that can present as ALF. It can also be considered an acute-on-chronic disease process that a patient may not have been aware of before hepatic failure.

Vascular

Vascular causes of ALF include portal vein thrombosis, Budd-Chiari syndrome (hepatic vein thrombosis), venoocclusive disease, ischemic disease, hepatic artery thrombosis (especially post transplant), and ischemic hepatitis (seen in the setting of severe hypotension or recent hepatic tumor chemoembolization).[7]

Malignancy

Malignancy infiltration may also be a cause of ALF. This may be caused by a primary liver tumor or a secondary tumor.

HEPATIC ENCEPHALOPATHY

Hepatic encephalopathy is brain dysfunction directly related to liver disease. It can range from mild to a comatose state. Grading of encephalopathy is important when evaluating patients with ALF because patients with lower grades of encephalopathy are more likely to have spontaneous recovery (**Table 1**).[6,7]

DIAGNOSIS

Rapid recognition of ALF and rapid diagnosis are the key to survival. Any patient with new-onset altered mental status and an INR greater than 1.5 (absent anticoagulation) needs admission to the hospital for further work-up. Given the possible rapid evolution of ALF, early transfer or admission to an ICU should be considered.[6] History taking should show careful attention to viral exposure and possible drug or chemical exposure. Physical examination should specifically look for stigmata of chronic liver disease because the treatment pathway for these patients is quite different. During the physical examination, specific attention to the neurologic status should be made to gauge the presence and degree of hepatic encephalopathy.

Initial laboratory examination should be directed toward causes of ALF as well as determining how critical the illness is. At minimum, laboratory examination should include[9]

INR
Basic metabolic panel
Magnesium, phosphorus, amylase, and lipase
Aspartate aminotransferase, alanine aminotransferase, alkaline phosphatase,
    γ-glutamyltransferase, total bilirubin, albumin
Arterial blood gas
Arterial lactate

Table 1
Grading of hepatic encephalopathy

Grade	Level of Consciousness	Personality and Intellect	Neurologic Signs	Electroencephalogram Abnormalities
0	Normal	Normal	Normal	None
Subclinical	Normal	Normal	Abnormality only in psychometric test	None
1	Day/night sleep reversal, restlessness	Forgetfulness, mild confusion, agitation, irritability	Tremor, apraxia, incoordination, impaired handwriting	Triphasic waves (5 Hz)
2	Lethargy, slowed responses	Disorientation to time, loss of inhibition, inappropriate behavior	Asterixis, dysarthria, hypoactive reflexes	Triphasic waves (5 Hz)
3	Somnolence, Confussion	Disorientation to place, aggressive behavior	Asterixis, muscular rigidity, Babinski signs, hyperactive reflexes	Triphasic waves (5 Hz)
4	Coma	None	Decerebration	Delta/slow wave activity

Data from Sood GK. eMedicine for WebMD: acute liver failure: treatment and medication. Updated online. Available at: http://emedicine.medscape.com. Accessed June 25, 2009.

Complete blood count
Blood type and screen
Acetaminophen level
Toxicology screen
Viral hepatitis serologies, including anti–hepatitis A virus IgM, hepatitis B surface
    antigen, anti–hepatitis B core antibody, anti–hepatitis D virus, anti–hepatitis E
    virus, and anti–hepatitis C virus
Ceruloplasmin
Pregnancy test (women)
Ammonia
Antinuclear antibody, anti–smooth muscle antibody, immunoglobulin levels
HIV status.

Radiology studies vary on presentation. Doppler ultrasound of the liver helps rule out Budd-Chiari syndrome. CT or MRI of the liver is frequently used to rule out hepatocellular carcinoma or other cancers as well as to examine the liver for signs of cirrhosis. CT of the head is helpful to rule out lesion or mass effect, which may provide an alternate explanation for a decreased mental status other than hepatic encephalopathy. Of note, the head CT is not sensitive for assessing cerebral edema due to intracranial hypertension in acute liver failure.

TREATMENT

Treatment varies by cause. In general, supportive measures and correcting metabolic disorders are the mainstay of treatment. Treatment of ALF patients requires a team approach. Critical care, transplant medicine, hepatology, neurology, neurosurgery, and infectious disease may all play a role in the management of patients.

Generally, there are several decision points during the treatment course of ALF patients. The first is admission to an ICU. Patients with grade II encephalopathy should be admitted to an ICU.[10] When encephalopathy reaches grade III, a decompressive nasogastric tube should be placed and intubation strongly considered.[11] Once a patient is intubated, the clinician loses the ability to monitor worsening encephalopathy. Many centers use intracranial pressure (ICP) monitoring to measure and treat rising ICP levels; however, the use of ICP monitoring is controversial.[12] Given the varied preferences, this leads to the second decision point. Once a patient has reached grade II encephalopathy, consultation with a transplant center is advised.[6]

General ICU management[11]
    Neurologic
        Sedation should be avoided if possible to ensure adequate mental status
            checks
        Elevate the head of bed 30°
        Consider ICP monitoring and management in the setting of elevated intracranial
            pressure (defined as >20 mm hg), pharmacologic interventions include os-
            motherapy in the form of Mannitol and Hypertonic Saline, Hypothermia and
            Barbituate coma.
    Renal failure
        If there is an indication for Renal Replacement therapy, consider continuous ve-
            novenous filtration if the patient is hemodynamically stable since intermittent
            hemodialysis has been associated with sudden rises in intracranial hyperten-
            sion and herniation due to fluid shifts.

Cardiovascular

    Monitory hemodynamics to keep patient normotensive. Hypotension and hypertension should be avoided. Consider a Swan-Ganz catheter to assess volume status.

Coagulopathy[13]

    In the absence of bleeding, it is not necessary to correct coagulopathy. Consider correction with fresh frozen plasma for procedures or when coagulopathy is extreme (INR >7).

    In patients who are nonresponsive to fresh frozen plasma, consider recombinant factor VIIa.

    Platelet transfusions can be used for platelet less than 20 k or PLT less than 50 when procedures are necessary. Cryoprecipitate in the setting of bleeding if Fibrinogen is less than 100.

The Role of N-Acetylcysteine in ALF

Although N-acetylcysteine (NAC) has been the mainstay in the treatment of acetaminophen overdose, recent studies have also shown its effectiveness in decreasing mortality in nonacetaminophen overdoses.[14] Given the benefits of NAC, it should be started as soon as possible on any ALF patient.

Specific Treatments

Acetaminophen

NAC is the mainstay of treatment of ALF from acetaminophen toxicity. Oral and IV forms are equally efficacious; however, encephalopathy and nausea generally make the IV form preferred in the late stage.[15] Although NAC should be started as soon as possible, there is increased survival even if started late in the treatment course.[16] Activated charcoal can also be used early in the treatment course.

Mushroom poisoning

Although evidence is contradictory, current guidelines recommend penicillin and silibin (milk thistle) as treatment for mushroom poisoning.[17]

Autoimmune hepatitis

Some patients may respond to steroid therapy (40–60 mg/d of prednisone or equivalent).[18]

Viral hepatitis

Acyclovir is the recommended therapy for ALF caused by herpes simplex virus .[19]

   Hepatitis B may be treated with nucleoside analogs although this remains controversial.[20]

Vascular insults

Budd-Chiari syndrome may be treated with transhepatic portal shunt.[21]

Liver Transplantation for ALF

Ultimately, liver transplantation remains the ultimate treatment of ALF. Ultimately, the decision to transplant is dependent on the probability for recovery without transplant. In general the three major predictors of recovery are degree of encephalopathy, age, and the cause of ALF. Grade I-II encephalopathy has a 70% to 80% rate of spontaneous recovery, whereas grade IV has less than a 20% rate of spontaneous recovery. Similarly, age less than 10 years or greater than 40 years is a poor predictor for

Table 2
King's College criteria for liver transplantation in ALF

Acetaminophen Hepatotoxicity	Nonacetaminophen ALF
Arterial lactate >3.5–4 h after resuscitation OR	Arterial lactate >3.5 4 h after resuscitation OR
pH <7.30 or arterial lactate >3.012 h after resuscitation OR	INR >6.5 (PT >100 s) OR
INR >6.5 (PT >100 s)	Any of the 3 of the following: INR >3.5 (PT >50 s)
Stage 3 or 4 encephalopathy	Age <10 or >40 y Serum bilirubin >17.5 mg/dL
Serum creatinine >3.4 mg/dL	Duration of jaundice >7 d
	Etiology: drug reaction

spontaneous recovery.[22] Finally, acetaminophen overdose, hepatitis A, and hepatitis B have a greater rate of spontaneous recovery than other causes.[23]

Several statistical models have been advanced for the prediction of spontaneous recovery in ALF. The King's College Criteria is the most commonly used (**Table 2**)[22]:

Sensitivity for King's College Criteria is approximately 90%. Criticism revolves around the specificity, which has been shown to be approximately 70%.[24] Despite this, no other model has demonstrated greater operating characteristics.[25]

The decision to list patients for transplant is a complex one. It revolves around limited resources, examination of patients' social support, and their ability to comply with complicated medical regimens. Evaluating these criteria in the face of an unconscious, rapidly deteriorating patient makes the challenge even more difficult. A multidisciplinary group, including social workers, transplant surgeons, hepatologists, and anesthesia and other providers, must be available to rapidly assess patients.

Once a decision has been made to list a patient, the patient is placed on the transplant list as status 1A. This allocates the first appropriate liver in a center's United Network for Organ Sharing region to the patient.[26] Overall, the survival rate of patients transplanted for ALF is excellent and equals that of patients transplanted for other causes.[2] Some studies have found, however, a higher death rate for patients listed, suggesting regional variation.[27]

SUMMARY

Overall rates of survival for ALF have improved substantially in the past 15 years. Although liver transplantation is somewhat responsible for the improved survival rate, it comes during a time of increased research in the critical care and hepatology arenas.

REFERENCES

1. Hoofnagle JH, Carithers RL, Sapiro C, et al. Fulminant hepatic failure: summary of a workshop. Hepatology 1995;21:240–52.
2. Ostapowicz GA, Fontana RJ, Schiodt FV, et al. Results of a prospective study of acute liver failure at 17 tertiary care centers in the United States. Ann Intern Med 2002;137:947–54.
3. 2008 Annual report of the U.S. Organ procurement and transplantation network and the scientific registry of transplant recipients: transplant data

1998–2007. U.S. Department of Health and Human Services. Health Resources and Services Administration. Healthcare Systems Bureau. Division of Transplantation. Rockville (MD).

4. Gotthardt D, Riediger C, Weiss KH, et al. Fulminant hepatic failure: etiology and indications for liver transplantation [review]. Nephrol Dial Transplant 2007; 22(Suppl 8):viii5–8.

5. Trey C, Davidson C. The management of fulminant hepatic failure. In: Popper H, Schaffner F, editors. Progress in liver disease. New York: Grune and Stratton; 1970. p. 282.

6. Polson J, Lee WM. AASLD position paper: the management of acute liver failure. Hepatology 2005;41:1179–97.

7. Goldberg E, Chopra S. Up to date: acute liver failure: definition; etiology; and prognostic indicators. Available at: http://www.uptodate.com. Accessed November 5, 2009.

8. Sood GK. eMedicine for WebMD: acute liver failure: treatment and medication. Available at: http://www.emedicine.medscape.com. Accessed June 25, 2009.

9. Lee WM, Schiodt FV. Fulminant hepatic failure. In: Schiff ER, Sorrell MF, Maddrey WC, editors. Schiff's diseases of the liver. 10th edition. Baltimore (MD): Lippincott Williams & Wilkins; 2006. p. 1623–9.

10. Stravitz RT, Kramer AH, Davern T, et al. Acute Liver Failure Study Group Intensive care of patients with acute liver failure: recommendations of the U.S. Acute Liver Failure Study Group. Crit Care Med 2007;35(11):2498–508.

11. Bernal W. Intensive care support therapy. Liver Transpl 2003;9(9):S15–7.

12. Lidofsky SD, Bass NM, Prager MC, et al. Intracranial pressure monitoring and liver transplantation for fulminant hepatic failure. Hepatology 1992;16:1–7.

13. Pereira SP, Langley PG, Williams R. The management of abnormalities of hemostasis in acute liver failure. Semin Liver Dis 1996;16(4):403–14.

14. Lee WM, Hynan LS, Rossaro L, et al. Acute Liver Failure Study Group. Intravenous N-acetylcysteine improves transplant-free survival in early stage non-acetaminophen acute liver failure. Gastroenterology 2009;137:856–64.

15. Vale JA, Proudfoot AT. Paracetamol (acetaminophen) poisoning. Lancet 1995; 346:547–52.

16. Harrison PM, Keays R, Bray GP, et al. Improved outcome of paracetamol-induced fulminant hepatic failure by late administration of acetylcysteine. Lancet 1990; 335:1572–3.

17. Moroni F, Fantozzi R, Masini E, et al. A trend in therapy of Amanita phalloides poisoning. Arch Toxicol 1976;36:111–5.

18. Czaja AJ, Freese DK. AASLD Practice guidelines: diagnosis and treatment of autoimmune hepatitis. Hepatology 2002;36:479–97.

19. Peters DJ, Greene WH, Ruggiero F, et al. Herpes simplex-induced fuminant hepatitis in adults: a call for empiric therapy. Dig Dis Sci 2000;45:2399–404.

20. Tillmann HL, Hadem J, Leifeld L, et al. Safety and efficacy of lamivudine in patients with severe acute or fulminant hepatitis B, a multicenter experience. J Viral Hepat 2006;13:256–63.

21. Murad SD, Valla DC, de Groen PC, et al. Determinants of survival and the effect of portosystemic shunting in patients with Budd-Chiari syndrome. Hepatology 2004; 39:500–8.

22. O'Grady JG, Alexander GJ, Hayllar KM, et al. Early indicators of prognosis in fulminant hepatic failure. Gastroenterology 1989;97:439–45.

23. White H. Evaluation and management of liver failure. In: Rippe J, editor. Intensive care medicine. Boston: Little Brown; 1996. p. 1733–8.

24. Anand A, Nightingale P, Neuberger J. Early indicators of prognosis in fulminant hepatic failure: an assessment of the King's criteria. J Hepatol 1997;26(1): 62–8.

25. Shakil AO, Kramer D, Mazariegos GV, et al. Acute liver failure: clinical features, outcome analysis, and applicability of prognostic criteria. Liver Transpl 2000;6: 163–9.

26. García-Gil FA, Luque P, Ridruejo R, et al. Liver transplant in emergency 0 (UNOS status 1). Transplant Proc 2006;38(8):2465–7.

27. Bismuth H, Samuel D, Castaing D, et al. Orthotopic liver transplantation in fulminant and subfulminant hepatitis. The Paul Brousse experience. Ann Surg 1995; 222:109–19.

Liver Transplant Considerations for Evaluation, CTP, and MELD

Sharon B. Mathews, MS, RN, CPTC[a], Wanda Allison, RN, BSN, CCTC[b],
Sonia Lin, PharmD, BCPS[c,d],*

KEYWORDS

- MELD • Pretransplant evaluation • Liver evaluation
- Waitlist mortality • Transplant survival

Liver transplantation has been available as a viable therapeutic option for patients with fulminant liver failure and end-stage liver disease since the early 1980s. Only since 1987 has a more formal liver allocation system, and an allocation system for all other solid organs, been put into place through the establishment of the Organ Procurement and Transplantation Network (OPTN).[1] Liver transplantation is associated with an overall decreased risk of mortality, and these mortality benefits increase with severity of liver disease.[2] In addition, liver transplantation is associated with significantly lower morbidity, as measured by hospital admission rates and average length of stay, compared with staying on the waiting list.[3]

Currently, more than 16,000 candidates are on the waiting list for a liver transplant (based on OPTN data as of June 18, 2010). Before being listed, all patients are required to undergo a detailed evaluation by various members of a multidisciplinary transplant team to assess candidacy for transplantation. Aspects of this evaluation include establishing the cause of liver disease, determining presence of cirrhosis complications, determining presence of contraindications to transplantation, and completing a comprehensive psychosocial evaluation.[4] This article reviews the

---

[a] Transplant Services, UMass Memorial Medical Center, 55 Lake Avenue North, Worcester, MA 01655, USA
[b] Clinical Operations & Services, Emory Liver Transplant Program, Emory Healthcare, 1365 Clifton Road, NE, Atlanta, GA 30052, USA
[c] Department of Pharmacy Practice, College of Pharmacy, University of Rhode Island, 41 Lower College Road, Fogarty Hall, Room 27, Kingston, RI 02881, USA
[d] Department of Pharmacy, UMass Memorial Medical Center, 55 Lake Avenue North, Worcester, MA 01655, USA
* Corresponding author. Department of Pharmacy Practice, College of Pharmacy, University of Rhode Island, 41 Lower College Road, Fogarty Hall, Room 27, Kingston, RI 02881.
E-mail address: SLin@uri.edu

Crit Care Nurs Clin N Am 22 (2010) 403–411
doi:10.1016/j.ccell.2010.05.002   ccnursing.theclinics.com
0899-5885/10/$ – see front matter © 2010 Elsevier Inc. All rights reserved.

process involved in evaluating patients to establish listing suitability for liver transplantation, and how livers are allocated after patients are placed on the waitlist.

As of October 2009, 129 deceased-donor liver transplant programs are available in the US. These programs are often housed in level one trauma centers in large cities, and are tertiary referral centers where patients from the local, regional, or multistate areas may be referred for transplant evaluation. Although located in diverse parts of the country, many similarities exist among these transplant programs. One of the more apparent is the complex evaluation process to determine transplant candidacy. In the US, all transplant programs, regardless of size or annual volumes, must adhere to the same national standards and regulations.

Health care is well known to be a regulated industry; similarly, solid organ transplantation within the health care industry is also carefully regulated. National agencies that govern, oversee, and monitor transplantation include the Department of Transplantation under the Health Resources and Service Administration (HRSA) of the US Department of Health and Human Services (DHHS), the United Network for Organ Sharing (UNOS), the OPTN, Centers for Medicare and Medicaid Services (CMS), the Joint Commission, and individual State Departments of Public Health (DPH). UNOS is contracted by the US. DHHS to promote and scientifically advance organ procurement and transplantation on a national scale throughout the United States. More recently, each transplant center may have a compliance officer assigned to transplant, or a dedicated transplant staff member whose role is to provide ongoing evidence (eg, documentation) that the program remains compliant with all of the multiagency requirements. Continuous review of center-specific processes ensures the best possible outcomes for patients and maximizes every organ that becomes available for transplantation.

The liver transplant evaluation is a multidisciplinary process. After the initial referral and confirmation of a patient's insurance information, a Transplant Financial Coordinator (or Counselor) (TFC) will then complete all necessary forms to obtain an insurance authorization so the patient may come to the transplant center for pretransplant evaluation. Some insurance companies administer what is termed a *blanket* or global *authorization* for transplantation. This authorization covers all previously disclosed laboratory tests, noninvasive and invasive testing, and annual age- and gender-specific screening tests that are required of all potential transplant candidates. If a patient's insurance company does not offer this benefit, the TFC will complete documentation, forward it to the patient's insurance company, and wait a prescribed amount of time for the Pre-Transplant Authorization for Evaluation to be approved and returned to the center. Once the authorization is in place, the patient may be scheduled for their initial appointment at the transplant center.

Every potential transplant candidate must meet and interact with a multidisciplinary team consisting of physicians (this may include the transplant surgeon, transplant hepatologist, anesthesiologist, and interventional radiologist), transplant social workers, transplant nurse, coordinators, dieticians, and any other necessary health care team members deemed appropriate per the transplant center. The potential candidate's medical and psychosocial health is assessed for suitability for transplant consideration.[5]

Potential transplant candidates are then required to undergo a rigorous battery of testing. This testing includes radiologic imaging, cardiac testing, pulmonary testing, routine age-appropriate cancer screening, immunizations, and extensive laboratory testing. After all testing and consultations are completed, the patient's case is discussed at a patient selection committee meeting. The selection committee is comprised of members of the multidisciplinary liver team. The potential recipient's candidacy for transplant is determined at this meeting. Possible recommendations from the committee include: approved for listing, further workup needed, not a candidate, or too early for transplant. The potential recipient is notified in writing of the outcome as outlined by the OPTN/UNOS and CMS regulations.[6]

The time frame required for the evaluation process to establish a patient's transplant candidacy, as well as the availability of donor livers, impacts upon the time to transplantation. In 2003, HRSA initiated the Organ Donation Breakthrough Collaborative (ODBC), with the support and cooperation of UNOS/OPTN and several other agencies. Prompted by the nationwide shortage of organs, one of the Collaborative's desired goals was to institute best practices in the nation's largest hospitals, thereby increasing the number of donor organs available for transplantation throughout the US.[7] A performance improvement approach model developed by the Institute for Healthcare Improvement (IHI) called the IHI Breakthrough Series, was implemented & utilized by the Collaborative participants.[8] This lead to an increase in the number of organs donated across the country over the next several months.

Building on the success of the ODBC, the Transplant Growth and Management Collaborative (TGMC) was established and supported by the DHHS. This Collaborative sought increased participation from the transplant centers, donor hospitals and organ procurement organizations (OPOs), together with key leaders from across the nation. The primary goal was to help increase the number of organs transplanted, thereby increasing the number of patients removed from the waitlist and decreasing the number of patients awaiting life-saving transplants. The TGMC devised a report entitled "Best Practice Evaluation," available to all participants on the World Wide Web.[9] A primary area of focus of this report was the actual number of days it takes for a potential candidate to move from referral to evaluation to actual listing on the national deceased donor waitlist for liver transplantation. The TGMC challenged each participating center improve their patient evaluation process in order to meet or exceed the established goal of reducing their center's current referral-to-listing timeframe to half of the previous fiscal year's total. For example, if a transplant center's previous fiscal year's referral-to-listing timeframe was 136 days, the target for the current fiscal year would be 68 days. Although these data were only collected until August 2008 by the TGMC from each participating transplant center (verified by UNOS/OPTN), the final results showed substantial improvement from the reporting centers toward this end (Shannon Dowell, RN, personal communication, 2009).

Each transplant center is responsible for ensuring that the evaluation process for every potential transplant candidate is as smooth and expeditious as possible. Despite each center's best efforts, the timeframe from referral of potential candidates to placement of their name on the liver transplant waiting list varies among centers. Unfortunately, much disparity exists regarding each center's actual referral-to-listing process and the timeframe involved, because of the nonstandardization of definitions between centers. One center may categorize a referral date differently from another, thereby creating difficulty when trying to compare data points, especially for consumers.

TRANSPLANT PRIORITIZATION AFTER LISTING: MODEL FOR END STAGE LIVER DISEASE VERSUS CHILD-TURCOTTE-PUGH SCORES

Once patients are placed on the UNOS wait list as appropriate candidates for transplantation, a prioritization algorithm is followed to determine which patient will receive the next available deceased-donor liver. When the OPTN was first established,

Table 1
Child-Turcotte-Pugh score for severity of liver disease

Points	1	2	3
Subjective variables			
Ascites	None	Controlled	Not controlled
Hepatic encephalopathy	None	Controlled	Not controlled
Objective variables			
Bilirubin (mg/dL)	0–2	2–3	>3
Albumin (g/dL)	>3.5	2.8–3.5	<2.8
Prothrombin time (seconds prolonged)	0–3	4–6	>6

Child-Turcotte-Pugh class A, 5–6 (well compensated disease); class B, 7–9 (significant functional compromise); class C, ≥ 10 (decompensated disease).

allocation of deceased-donor livers was initially prioritized based on the acuity of illness; time accrued on the waiting list was also considered.[1] Severity of illness was reflected by the level of care, and thus the type of care setting patients required. Patients in an intensive care unit (ICU) were considered the sickest and thus received greatest priority. Patients who required hospitalization (other than ICU) were next in line in terms of priority, followed by patients who were able to receive care at home. However, criteria for admission to the hospital (non-ICU) or ICU care settings were not standardized and minimal listing criteria had not been established. This allocation method fell out of favor as the disparity between number of waitlisted patients and number of donor organs available for transplant widened.

The Child-Turcotte-Pugh (CTP) score was used exclusively in the OPTN liver allocation policy between January 19, 1998 and February 26, 2002 as a more standardized clinical assessment of illness severity.[10] This scoring system was originally developed by Child and Turcotte in 1964, and then modified by Pugh and colleagues[11] in 1973 to predict the outcome of patients with cirrhosis undergoing surgical treatment for portal hypertension, based on assessment of liver disease severity.[1,12] The CTP score incorporated the presence of cirrhosis complications and more objective measures of liver dysfunction (**Table 1**).[13] A CTP score of seven or greater was the minimal requirement for listing.

Once placed on the wait list, patients with chronic liver disease were then prioritized into three categories of medical urgency based on their CTP score, in order of decreasing priority (**Table 2**).[1] Patients who did not meet any of these criteria were prioritized based upon their wait time. A separate status 1 category was implemented

Table 2
Waiting list prioritization

Status	Criteria
1	Fulminant hepatic failure, primary graft nonfunction, hepatic artery thrombosis within 7 days posttransplantation, acute decompensated Wilson's disease
2A	CTP score ≥ 10 AND <7 days predicted survival
2B	CTP score ≥ 10 or CTP score ≥ 7 AND major complications of portal hypertension
3	CTP score ≥ 7

Data from Freeman RB, Wiesner RH, Roberts JP, et al. Improving liver allocation: MELD and PELD. Am J Transplant 2004;4(Suppl 9):115.

in 1997 for adult liver transplant candidates and was comprised of patients who presented with acute hepatic failure for various predetermined causes. These patients exemplified the most medically urgent patients awaiting liver transplantation.

The application of the CTP allocation system represented an improvement over previous allocation strategies. However, reliance on the CTP score and wait time also had its limitations. The elements of ascites and hepatic encephalopathy in the CTP score are subjective by nature. Interpretations of the score vary among clinicians, and its assessment is subject to manipulation with medications such as diuretics and lactulose. Also, the CTP score has not been widely validated to predict mortality of patients on the waiting list, and the time on the waiting list does not accurately reflect medical urgency for transplantation.[1,12]

The Model for End Stage Liver Disease (MELD) scoring system (previously known as the Mayo End-Stage Liver Disease model) has replaced the CTP score as the basis for liver allocation in the United States. Although both the CTP and MELD scoring systems reflect waitlist mortality and thus medical urgency or need for transplantation, the MELD score eliminates the subjective element of the CTP score.[14] The MELD score incorporates three objective biochemical variables related to liver disease: serum creatinine, bilirubin, and prothrombin time. The original MELD equation, which included cause of cirrhosis as the fourth variable, was initially developed by the Mayo Clinic to predict the short-term prognosis of patients undergoing a transjugular intrahepatic portosystemic shunt (TIPS) procedure.[15] Its application in the chronic liver disease population was later validated for predicting 3-month mortality, including patients with compensated or decompensated liver cirrhosis and those with cholestatic liver disease. Incorporation of cause of liver disease did not improve the 3-month mortality predictability, and therefore was eventually left out of the model (**Fig. 1**).[13]

The Pediatric End-stage Liver Disease (PELD) score is a similar model to MELD that was developed from data representative of a cross-section of children awaiting liver transplantation. Variables incorporated into the PELD score include age, albumin, bilirubin, prothrombin time, and growth failure. This model was also validated to predict 3-month mortality and was implemented for liver allocation to pediatric recipients, ages 0 to 17 years in 2002.[1]

HEPATOCELLULAR CARCINOMA

Despite wide applicability of the MELD score, it does not adequately reflect the prognosis for some liver diseases, particularly hepatocellular carcinoma (HCC). Patients with stage I and II HCC have a higher risk of tumor progression that exceeds their

---

Original MELD score
$$MELD = [0.957 \times Ln\,(creatinine) + 0.378 \times Ln\,(bilirubin) + 1.12 \times Ln\,(INR) + 0.643] + 0.643 \times (cause\ of\ cirrhosis)$$

OPTN/UNOS MELD score
$$MELD = [0.957 \times Ln\,(creatinine^{**}) + 0.378 \times Ln\,(bilirubin^{**}) + 1.12 \times Ln\,(INR^{**})] + 0.643]$$

PELD score
$$PELD = (0.436 \times age^{a}) - (0.687 \times log\,(albumin)) + (0.480 \times log\,(bilirubin)) + (1.857 \times log\,(INR)) + (0.667 \times growth\ failure\,)$$

*Cholestatic liver disease = 0; all others = 1
**Values < 1.0 rounded up to 1.0
^{a}Age < 1 year = 1; all others = 0
^{b}Values > 2 standard deviations from the norm = 1; all others = 0

Fig. 1. Model for End Stage Liver Disease and Pediatric End-stage Liver Disease scores. (*From* Freeman RB, Wiesner RH, Roberts JP, et al. Improving liver allocation: MELD and PELD. Am J Transplant 2004;4(Suppl 9):116; with permission.)

risk of death. In addition, if their disease has spread (ie, is metastatic), these patients become ineligible for liver transplantation altogether. The liver allocation policy was updated to account for this; exceptional MELD scores of 24 and 29 were initially assigned to patients with stage I and II HCC, respectively.[1] These scores were later lowered to corresponding MELD scores of 20 and 24 in 2003, because of comparatively higher mortality rates observed in patients who did not have HCC with similar MELD scores.[1,16]

However, this method of liver allocation for patients with HCC remains a controversial topic. The application of exception points provides an advantage to patients with HCC that may decrease the chances of otherwise sicker candidates receiving an organ in a timely fashion. The allocation policy was updated again in 2004 and the MELD exception was no longer assigned to patients with stage I HCC because of their relatively low risk of being removed from the list as a result of tumor progression.[1,17] This issue will likely continue to be controversial as the number of patients with liver disease caused by HCC continues to rise. The incidence of HCC in the United States has doubled over the past 20 years.[18] UNOS Policy 3.6.4.4, "Liver Transplant Candidates with Hepatocellular Carcinoma (HCC)," is very prescriptive vis-à-vis the MELD point system. The most recent policy revision was accepted in June 2009.[19]

In general, HCC surveillance on all pretransplant patients consists of a serum alpha-fetoprotein (AFP) and an ultrasound, CT, or MRI scan is required every 3 months. For HCC detected in patients without cirrhosis or who have compensated cirrhosis, a resection or locoregional therapy is considered (consult made to interventional radiology). A chest CT or MRI is performed at diagnosis to evaluate for metastasis. If metastatic disease is found or suspected, further testing will be completed. Patients with confirmed metastatic disease are not eligible to undergo transplantation.

HCC in patients with decompensated cirrhosis denotes different therapy. If within Milan criteria,[20] an abdominal CT or MRI is performed every 3 months with serum AFP obtained. Potential candidates will proceed with orthotopic liver transplantation evaluation and listing pending approval by the transplant center's selection committee. An interventional radiology consult is considered for locoregional therapy.

Monitoring patients with HCC is labor-intensive for the transplant center's pretransplant liver coordinator. Compliance with center-specific protocols and regulated data-specific requirements is mandatory. An error or omission of required tests and accompanying documentation may result in disciplinary action or the potential loss of certification as a transplant center.[19]

FULMINANT HEPATIC FAILURE

Fulminant hepatic failure (FHF), also known as *acute liver failure*, is a disease entity that does not lend itself to, and is thus an exception from, the MELD scoring system. Patients are classified as having FHF if they show acute hepatic deterioration, defined as the progression from the onset of jaundice to the development of hepatic encephalopathy within an 8-week period, in the absence of chronic liver disease. The most common causes of FHF include acetaminophen toxicity, hepatitis non-A or E, drug-induced causes, hepatitis B, and hepatitis A.[21] This type of liver failure more commonly affects younger individuals in previously good health and is associated with an 80% to 90% mortality rate if left untreated. Conversely, survival rates of 90% have been shown with liver transplantation as a treatment option.[4]

Each center has specific management algorithms for patients with FHF. These patients may present to the emergency department or outpatient clinic with vague flu-like symptoms, such as anorexia and malaise. Typically, liver function tests are only ordered after jaundice appears, revealing abnormally elevated bilirubin, aspartate aminotransferase, alanine aminotransferase, and prothrombin time/international normalized ratio. These patients must be carefully monitored in a hospital setting because they may progress to advanced stages of encephalopathy (3 or 4) requiring intubation for airway protection. Initial evaluation consists of laboratory values, including serologies; arterial blood gases are obtained. Abdominal imaging is performed to determine vessel patency.

Once the potential recipient is evaluated by the liver transplant team, the transplant coordinator is notified to begin an immediate inpatient evaluation and listing. If cardiac imaging is needed, a transesophageal echocardiogram at bedside is ordered. This type of expedited review and workup is performed in ICUs across the United States. What experts know and work diligently to achieve is a liver transplant for patients experiencing FHF, because liver transplantation is currently the best therapeutic option for irreversible liver failure.[4]

OTHER MELD EXCEPTIONS

Other rare diagnoses and exceptional situations that warrant a higher assigned MELD score can be presented to a regional peer-review board (RRB) for consideration. These scenarios include, but are not limited to, patients with hepatic artery thrombosis after liver transplantation, refractory upper gastrointestinal and variceal bleeding requiring transfusions or Blakemore tube insertions, hepatopulmonary syndrome, portopulmonary hypertension, primary oxaluria, familial amyloid polyneuropathy, inborn errors of metabolism, and severe polycystic liver disease.[12,22,23] MELD exceptions for these disease states can range from automatic assignment of priority for liver transplantation, to additional MELD points applied based on predefined criteria, to requirement for application to an RRB for exception consideration.[23]

SUMMARY

The detailed evaluation of a patient for liver transplant candidacy involves health care professionals from various disciplines to ensure that liver transplantation is optimal for patient morbidity and mortality from the medical and psychosocial perspective. The national liver allocation policy is complex and should be updated periodically based on continual assessment of outcomes that result from current policies. Streamlining of policies and procedures and implementing appropriate documentation across all transplant centers is required and regulated by national agencies, such as OPTN/UNOS and CMS. This ensures safe and appropriate organ allocation and the delivery of high-quality transplant services.

REFERENCES

1. Freeman RB, Wiesner RH, Roberts JP, et al. Improving liver allocation: MELD and PELD. Am J Transplant 2004;4(Suppl 9):114–31.
2. Merion RM, Schaubel DE, Dykstra DM, et al. The survival benefit of liver transplantation. Am J Transplant 2005;5:307–13.
3. Schaubel DE, Wei G, Dykstra DM, et al. Hospitalization patterns before and after liver transplantation. Transplantation 2007;84:1590–4.
4. Koffron A, Stein JA. Liver transplantation: indications, pretransplant evaluation, surgery, and posttransplant complications. Med Clin North Am 2008;92: 861–88.

5. CMS Conditions of Participation, Section 42 FR §482.68-§482.104. Available at: http://www.cms.hhs.gov/CFCsAndCoPs/11_transplantcenter. Accessed October 1, 2009.

6. Federal Register/Vol. 72, No. 61/Friday, March 30, 2007 Rules and regulations. Available at: http://www.cms.hhs.gov/CertificationandComplianc/Downloads/Transplantfinal.pdf. Accessed October 1, 2009.

7. U.S. Department of Health and Human Services. Health resources and service administration knowledge gateway. The Organ Donation and Transplantation Community of Practice. Available at: http://www.healthdisparities.net/hdc/html/collaboratives.topics.tgmc.aspx. Accessed October 1, 2009.

8. US Department of Health and Human Services. Health resources and service administration, OPTN, news: breakthrough collaborative met with enthusiasm. Available at: http://optn.transplant.hrsa.gov/news/newsDetail.asp?id=307. Accessed October 1, 2009.

9. HRSA Transplant Center Growth and Management Collaborative. Best practices evaluation final report. U.S. Department of Health and Human Services, Health Resources and Services Administration, Healthcare Systems Bureau, Division of Transplantation. Available at: http://www.healthdisparities.net/hdc/hdcsearch/isysquery/15ae0fb7-2dd5-4b2f-a008-e5643507a3c1/1/doc/. September 2007. Accessed October 19, 2009.

10. United Network for Organ Sharing. Resources: Glossary. Available at: http://www.unos.org/esources/glossary.asp#C. Accessed September 24, 2009.

11. Pugh RN, Murray-Lyon IM, Dawson JL, et al. Transection of the oesophagus for bleeding oesophageal varices. Br J Surg 1973;60(8):646–9.

12. Cholongotas E, Marelli L, Shusang V, et al. A systematic review of the performance of the Model for End-Stage Liver Disease (MELD) in the setting of liver transplantation. Liver Transpl 2006;12:1049–61.

13. Weisner RH, McDiarmid SV, Kamath PS, et al. MELD and PELD: application of survival models to liver allocation. Liver Transpl 2001;7(7):567–80.

14. Schaubel DE, Guidinger MK, Biggins SW, et al. Survival benefit-based deceased-donor liver allocation. Am J Transplant 2009;9(Pt 2):970–81.

15. Malinchoc M, Kamath PS, Gordan FD, et al. A model to predict poor survival in patients undergoing transjugular intrahepatic portosystemic shunts. Heptatology 2000;31:864–71.

16. United Network for Organ Sharing. OPTN/UNOS board of directors meeting: executive summary of the minutes, Nov 2002. Available at: www.unos.org/SharedContentDocuments/Executive_Summary_Nov._2002.pdf. Accessed October 1, 2009.

17. Martin AP, Bartels M, Hauss J, et al. Overview of the MELD score and the UNOS adult liver allocation system. Transplant Proc 2007;39:3169–74.

18. El-Serag HB. Hepatocellular carcinoma: recent trends in the United States. Gastroenterology 2004;127:S27–34.

19. OPTN/UNOS Policy Organ Distribution. Allocation of livers. Available at: http://optn.transplant.hrsa.gov/PoliciesandBylaws2/policies/pdfs/policy_8.pdf. Accessed October 12, 2009.

20. Mazzaferro V, Ragalia E, Doci R, et al. Liver transplantation for the treatment of small hepatocellular carcinomas in patients with cirrhosis. N Engl J Med 1996; 334(11):693–9.

21. Schiodt FV, Atillasoy E, Shakil AO, et al. Etiology and outcome for 295 patients with acute liver failure in the United States. Liver Transpl Surg 1999;5(1):29–34.

22. Berg CL, Steffick DE, Edwards EB, et al. Liver and intestine transplantation in the United States 1998–2007. Am J Transplant 2009;9(Pt 2):907–31.
23. Freeman RB, Gish RG, Harper A, et al. Model for end-stage liver disease (MELD) exception guidelines: Results and recommendation from the MELD Exception Study Group and Conference (MESSAGE) for the approval of patients who need liver transplantation with diseases not considered by the standard MELD formula. Liver Transpl 2006;12(12 Suppl 3):S128–36.

Index

Note: Page numbers of article titles are in **boldface** type.

A

Acarbose, for hepatic encephalopathy, 346

Acute liver failure (ALF), **395–401**. See also *Fulminant hepatic failure (FHF).*
    bleeding complications of, 316
    causes of, 396
    coagulopathy in, **315–321**
        assessment of, 315–316
        cryoprecipitate for, 319
        fresh frozen plasma for, 318
        plasmapheresis for, 319
        recombinant factor VIIa for, 319
    course of, 395
    defined, 395
    diagnosis of, laboratory examination for, 397–398
        radiology studies for, 398
    gastrointestinal bleeding in, 316
    hemorrhage in, intracranial, 316
        spontaneous, 316
    hepatic encephalopathy in, 397–398
    invasive interventions for, hemodynamic monitoring, 317
        ICP monitoring, 318
        renal replacement therapy access, 317–318
    liver transplantation for, 399–400
    treatment of, ICU management, 398–399
        N-acetylcysteine in, 399
        specific, 399

Aeromonas species, infectious disease from, 296

Age, drug-induced liver disease and, 324

Antibiotics, for hepatic encephalopathy, 344–345

Antimicrobial agents, for infectious disease management, 298–299

Arginine vasopressin infusion, for hepatorenal syndrome, 360

Ascites, alcohol use and, 306
    and spontaneous bacterial peritonitis, 293
    diagnosis of, laboratory evaluation of ascites fluid in, 311
    etiologies of, 309–310
    management of, **309–314**
    referral for liver transplantation, 313
    treatment of, diuretics, 312
        paracentesis, serial large volume, 312
        surgical peritoneovenous shunts, 313
        transjugular intrahepatic portosystemic shunt, 312
    viral hepatitis and, 306

Crit Care Nurs Clin N Am 22 (2010) 413–419
doi:10.1016/S0899-5885(10)00054-7
0899-5885/10/$ – see front matter © 2010 Elsevier Inc. All rights reserved.

ccnursing.theclinics.com

Moving?

Make sure your subscription moves with you!

To notify us of your new address, find your **Clinics Account Number** (located on your mailing label above your name), and contact customer service at:

Email: journalscustomerservice-usa@elsevier.com

800-654-2452 (subscribers in the U.S. & Canada)
314-447-8871 (subscribers outside of the U.S. & Canada)

Fax number: 314-447-8029

Elsevier Health Sciences Division
Subscription Customer Service
3251 Riverport Lane
Maryland Heights, MO 63043

*To ensure uninterrupted delivery of your subscription, please notify us at least 4 weeks in advance of move.

Printed in the United States
By Bookmasters

Printed in the United States
By Bookmasters